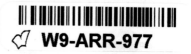

Ethical Dilemmas in Pediatrics

Edwin N. Forman   Rosalind Ekman Ladd

Ethical Dilemmas in Pediatrics

A Case Study Approach

Springer-Verlag
New York Berlin Heidelberg London
Paris Tokyo Hong Kong Barcelona

Edwin N. Forman, M.D.
Professor of Pediatrics, Brown
University, and Director, Pediatric
Hematology/Oncology, and
Coordinator, Pediatric Residency
Education, Rhode Island Hospital,
Providence, RI 02903, USA

Rosalind Ekman Ladd, Ph.D.
Professor of Philosophy,
Wheaton College, Norton, MA 02766;
and Lecturer in Pediatrics,
Brown University, and Affiliate Staff,
Rhode Island Hospital,
Providence, RI 02903, USA

Library of Congress Cataloging-in-Publication Data
Forman, Edwin N.
    Ethical dilemmas in pediatrics : a case study approach / Edwin N.
Forman, Rosalind Ekman Ladd.
        p.   cm.
    Includes bibliographical references and index.
    ISBN 0-387-97454-7 (alk. paper). — ISBN 3-540-97454-7 (alk.
paper)
        1. Pediatrics — Moral and ethical aspects — Case studies.   I. Ladd,
Rosalind Ekman.   II. Title.
    [DNLM: 1. Ethics, Medical — case studies.   2. Pediatrics — case
studies.   WS 21 F724e]
RJ47.F67   1991
174'.2 — dc20
DNLM/DLC
for Library of Congress   90-10398

Printed on acid-free paper.

Camera-ready copy provided by the authors.
Printed and bound by BookCrafters, Chelsea, Michigan.
Printed in the USA.

9 8 7 6 5 4 3 2 1

ISBN 0-387-97454-7 Springer-Verlag New York Berlin Heidelberg
ISBN 3-540-97454-7 Springer-Verlag Berlin Heidelberg New York

We wish to thank all the children from whose lives we have learned and the staff of the pediatric departments at Rhode Island Hospital and Women and Infants Hospital, from whose caring attitudes and challenging discussions we have benefited.

Preface

This book is addressed to all professionals concerned with the health care of children. It is, first and foremost, a teaching tool. It can be used for class discussion or case conferences with medical students or residents, nurses, and other staff in pediatrics or family medicine. It can also be used for self-teaching or continuing education by those already in practice.

No one who reads this book is a beginner at moral reasoning. However, many may well be beginners at discussions that focus sharply on the ethical issues in medicine and introduce philosophical analysis. The goal is to clarify, conceptualize, and guide reasoning in order to come to conclusions that can be defended with good reasons.

Case studies provide the most successful method of teaching medical ethics, posing the issues as they arise in real-life situations. The cases in this book are brief and rather skeletal in nature. This is partly to deflect the natural curiosity of those who are driven to seek more and more medical details, hoping thus to resolve the ethical issues or avoid them entirely. It also allows the reader to concentrate on one ethical issue at a time. In real life, of course, the hard questions arise often several at a time, embedded in a rich and complex medical and psychosocial background. As one must learn to walk before one can run, so it is wise to practice on cases where the key issue is highlighted.

The discussion questions following each case are, in a sense, the heart of the book, for the key to moral reasoning is knowing what questions to ask. The narrative following each case introduces vocabulary, distinctions, concepts, and analysis, designed only to guide the reader to a deeper understanding of the issues. In many cases no conclusion is reached, for in real life practitioners must reason out their own final clinical judgments, informed by both ethical considerations and scientific facts.

All the cases in this book are drawn from clinical experience, but with details changed to protect confidentiality. They range from the routine to the exotic, those that arise in hospital residency training and in office practice. These cases have constituted the substance of more than a decade of pediatric ethics rounds conducted by the authors in a major teaching hospital. We know they work: they challenge assumptions, make people think, provoke lively discussions. In short, they teach medical ethics.

Contents

Introduction

The Nature of Moral Reasoning

Clinical judgment involves moral reasoning, for health and wellbeing are highly prized human values, not just scientific facts. When there is consensus about values, moral reasoning may go unnoticed. When uncertainty or disagreement arises, then it becomes apparent that in a pluralistic society, different people hold different moral positions.

To practice good medicine, the value questions need to be addressed: it is important to recognize the ethical or value dimensions of clinical judgment, to have a conceptual framework in which to clarify and express the issues, to understand both sides of an issue, to recognize good reasons, and to understand the limits of ethics debates.

Socrates believed that knowledge, and especially moral reasoning, is not something that is poured into people, as if they were empty receptacles, but is something that is inherent in rational beings, waiting to be drawn forth, as a midwife draws forth the infant from the mother. This means that each person has the capability to do his or her own moral reasoning. In this sense, there are no moral experts and morality is not handed out by authorities. Instead, it is brought forth by a process of questioning, discussing, considering different points of view, and most importantly, looking for good reasons. It is an assumption of this book that moral reasoning is a skill that can be learned.

The fact that there are no moral experts and that, in a pluralistic society, one cannot expect that there will be a simple set of accepted values and one right answer makes the study of ethics very different from the study of science. Scientific questioning ends when the empirical data are in; an answer is accepted if it works.

Ethical disagreements, by contrast, may begin with different basic principles and end with people agreeing to disagree. However, this does not mean that anything goes. Moral reasoning is reasoning, and one must have good reasons to defend one's position on a controversial issue. One learns to recognize good reasons by engaging in discussion and debate, considering opposite views, questioning oneself and others.

A good reason, in the context of moral questions, provides not only an answer to a question but a reason for doing something. It provides both justification and motivation. This is perhaps a complicated way of saying that moral reasoning is not a mere intellectual exercise; it is part of practical reasoning, which results in action. The practice of medicine is practical in this same sense: it is applied science.

For a thoughtful person, knowing that something works in medicine is not enough; one wants to know why it works and how it works. The same is true for moral reasoning: one wants not only to be able to achieve agreement, but to know how and why the arguments work.

There are many payoffs for developing skills in moral reasoning. The first, of course, is to be able to answer one's own questions about how to act in perplexing situations. It is not possible to avoid the issues, and there is obvious advantage to thinking clearly and logically about emotionally laden problems. Second, only practitioners who really understand the reasoning on both sides of an issue can communicate effectively with patients, families, and each other.

The Moral Questions

Physicians could spend considerable time studying moral theory, but their business and busyness requires a more pragmatic approach. The key to analyzing and conceptualizing the moral reasoning demanded by clinical decision-making lies in knowing what questions to ask. The following three are derived from the most commonly used classical and modern theories about how to answer the practical question, "What should I do?"

1. What are the risks and benefits? This is also commonly expressed in terms of benefits and burdens, and is familiar in other contexts as cost/benefit analysis. The reason for asking this question is to assess the consequences of any proposed decision; consequences for whom, for how many, for how long? No act is wrong in itself: its moral value derives from its consequences. Popularly put, this is the theory that claims the end justifies the means. The general principle underlying these questions, which expresses the heart of John Stuart Mill's (1806–1873) utilitarianism, is that what one should do is try to maximize the benefits and minimize the harms for the greatest number of people. Part of this principle is captured in a recent interpretation of the Hippocratic dictum, "First help, but if not, at least do no harm."

2. What are the rights of the individuals involved? According to this theory the rights of individuals and minority groups must be respected, even if doing so does not contribute to the greatest good of the majority. Thus, this theory may be in direct conflict with utilitarianism. Modern society suffers from a kind of moral schizophrenia, in that part of public policy is derived from utilitarianism, but part of it is derived from the theory of rights. As individuals and as society, people must decide which principle to follow in particular situations, and much

public debate is at the level of theory in this sense. Rights theory, as developed by Immanuel Kant (1724–1804), emphasizes respect for the dignity of the individual, and many moral dilemmas revolve around conflicting rights and can be resolved only by establishing hierarchies of duties and obligations to the different parties.

3. Is there a just distribution of benefits and burdens? Concerns about justice and fairness are intended to bring into balance concerns about cost/benefit and rights, and to force consideration of the large social issues about the organization of systems of allocation and access to resources. As developed by the contemporary philosopher John Rawls, perfect fairness could be achieved only if all citizens, rational and self-interested, could convene to develop laws and regulations with absolutely no knowledge of what place they themselves would hold in the society. This would guarantee a system in which even the least advantaged person would be treated fairly, and it is the ideal against which all current and future systems should be measured.

Part I
Making Decisions:
Whose Choice?

CHAPTER 1

Parents' Rights

"It really is time to consider surgery. Six urinary infections in the last 12 months, and the tests show vesicoureteral reflux. This can be repaired with surgery, and she'll be as good as new."

"No, no surgery. Annie's only 8, and I know her father wouldn't agree to it."

"Well, we can't go on treating it with antibiotics. It will cause terrible problems for her in the future—hypertension, renal failure, lots of discomfort and even a shorter life span."

"No, no surgery. That's final."

What should the physician do when parents refuse standard care for their child?

Discussion Questions

1. What rights do parents have in making medical decisions for their children?

2. What is the moral basis of parents' rights? Why do parents, not others, have rights over children?

3. What are the legal and moral limits of parents' rights?

In the past few years, we have seen the question of parents' rights to make medical decisions for their children raised with dramatic intensity. It is the stuff of newspaper headlines and TV specials.

It began in 1975 with the case of Karen Ann Quinlan, whose parents had to plead with a judge to be allowed to remove ventilator support from their comatose daughter. The Chad Green case gained national attention in 1978, when the court appointed a legal guardian in the place of his parents to assure continuation of chemotherapy instead of the Laetrile and vitamin therapy they had chosen for him. The Baby Doe cases in 1982 were hotly and publicly debated and prompted an attempt by the federal government to take decision-making power away from parents who refused aggressive therapy for seriously handicapped newborns. Then in 1989 there was the father in Chicago who held hospital staff at bay with a shotgun while he unplugged the respirator from his nearly brain-dead young son.

Cases that gain public notoriety are not the everyday fare of the pediatrician's practice, yet the issue of the rights of parents lies at the heart of many everyday management decisions. The moral foundation of parents' rights as well as the limits society places on them need to be understood in order to operate effectively in the branch of medicine where the patient does not stand alone but is intimately linked—physically, legally, emotionally, and economically—with one or both parents.

The Rights of Parents

Suppose that the doctor is convinced that Annie should have surgery. Does she have the obligation to honor the parents' decision, even if she believes it is wrong? Given her greater medical knowledge, experience, and objectivity, does she have the right to continue to try to persuade, cajole, or even coerce Annie's parents to change their minds? If they remain adamant, should she consider appealing to a state agency or to the courts, as one would in cases of refusal of life-saving therapy? Why shouldn't parents be required to choose the best medical treatment for their child? Why should they be allowed the liberty to make mistakes at their child's expense?

Medical paternalism is the view that the doctor knows best and the patient (parents) should not be allowed to choose. The problem with this view is that it assumes that the only relevant factors are medical. It confuses medical knowledge, in which the physician is clearly superior, with knowledge of a person's own best interests, which may be based at least in part on personal values.

For example, in a simple case of choosing between liquid or capsule vitamins for a small child, the physician knows that they are equally effective but the pills are cheaper; the parent weighs the time and trouble to be sure that each pill is swallowed successfully as more burdensome than the extra cost. Values may be weighed differently by different families, and respect for pluralism in values cautions against an unexamined medical paternalism.

Thus, Annie's physician should try to discover the family's reasons for their choice in order to know whether it is owing to a difference in values as opposed to a lack of understanding of the medical facts.

The Foundation of Parents' Rights

The most basic and fundamental question is why parents' values may be imposed on the child; that is, why parents have the moral right to decide for their children.

Proxy consent is generally obtained from biological parents or legal guardians. Why parents are assumed to be proxies for their children is answered in part by historical precedent: rights of parents over children are grounded on the property rights of fathers. This idea gives parents a good deal of latitude to mold children as they see fit.

More popular reasons for recognizing parents as decision-makers are: 1) they are the ones charged by society with responsibility for the welfare and up-bringing of children, and responsibility for children requires having the rights for decision-making over them, 2) parents are the people who live most directly with the consequences of their child-rearing, and 3) they have a genetic tie to their children.

A pragmatic view is that parents make the best qualified decision-makers because they know the child best. The parents who are helping to form the child are in the best position to know his or her needs and wants. Sensitive parents observe minute changes in their children's physical and mental states and know almost intuitively what is right for them.

Finally, an even newer theoretical position is that the intimacy of family life is among the greatest personal values. The special relationship between parents and child can be achieved only by protecting it from interference by others.

Whether or not parents do make the best decision-makers has been disputed. Some argue that parents, especially under the emotional stress of sudden accident or serious illness, are incompetent to make decisions. Moreover, the existence of child abuse and neglect by parents is evidence that not all parents always act in the best interest of their children.

The Limits of Parents' Rights

The physician in this case believes that Annie's parents are not making the right decision for their child. She believes that there are limits to the autonomy or freedom of parents to choose for their children. What are the limits set by law and by society's moral standards?

Legally, there are certain things society has decided parents cannot choose. Their liberty is limited by such things as required vaccinations, required school attendance, and the various criteria for child abuse and neglect. Although there is wide latitude given to families to allow them to practice various religions and lifestyles, courts have intervened to protect children and not allowed refusal of standard medical treatment in life-threatening situations by Jehovah's Witnesses and Christian Scientist parents.

In less than life-threatening situations, for the reasons given above, society is more reluctant to intervene between parents and child. Thus, the physician could not count on a court requiring surgery for Annie against her parents' wishes. On the other hand, society's interest in healthy children seems to be leading to an increasing willingness to intervene more.

For example, currently courts are being asked to intervene to protect a fetus by requiring a caesarean section even without the woman's consent and to restrict the freedom of drug-using women during pregnancy to prevent the birth of so-called cocaine babies. Strict laws requiring report of even suspected abuse or neglect also reflect an apparent trend toward greater limits on parents' rights.

On the other hand, no one has ever required that parents make "the very best" choice, but only that they meet some acceptable standard.

Morally, good conscience requires the physician to pursue the idea of surgery for Annie, discussing it at each future office visit. Good communication requires her to be patient and to continue to give information, trying to elicit and understand and then respond to the parents' reasons for not choosing surgery. Good doctor-patient relationship requires that she not be coercive or condemnatory. Respect for parents' rights and their concern for their child offer hope that they will choose surgery if and when they become convinced that it is, indeed, the best medical treatment for their child. In a case such as this, where nonsurgery is not a life-threatening harm, it can be postponed safely. When the time comes that the child's life is threatened or serious and irreversible morbidity is likely, then the physician will rightly feel compelled to call in legal authorities.

CHAPTER 2

Consulting the Child

"But I don't want to stay in the hospital overnight, Dr. Hartman. It always ends up longer than you say, and anyway my ear doesn't even hurt that much."

"Benjie, let's go through it again. I explained to you what happens with a bad ear infection. It doesn't seem so bad to you now, but when I look into it with my light, I see all kinds of red. With your low white cell count, if I let you go home with it, it might get worse in the middle of the night. You wouldn't want to to have to come back here then, would you?"

"Oh, for heaven's sake, doctor, you've been at it for 20 minutes. Why bother with all that explanation? You know he has to be admitted, and we'll do it whether he agrees or not."

What are the reasons for trying to get a child's agreement for necessary medical treatment?

Discussion Questions

1. In general, should children be given a voice in decisions affecting them? If so, why?

2. Are children competent to make decisions for themselves?

3. Is it in the child's interest to be involved in decision-making?

It used to be said that children should be seen and not heard. Historically, children were considered chattel or property, completely under the control of their parents. In contrast to this, our generation has seen a real movement toward greater rights for children. Theories of child-rearing now describe parents' roles as including teaching, guiding, and encouraging the development of decision-making skills. Adults are encouraged to offer choices even to very young children when possible and to give reasons for decisions when choices are not possible. The influence of John Dewey is profound: he argued that children learn by problem solving and that the goals of education in this country should be to develop skills in making thoughtful decisions, in order to develop adults who will be good citizens in a participatory democracy. Although parents and physicians are still obviously authority figures, they should not operate in an autocratic way.

Why Consult the Child?

Dr. Hartman's conversation with Benjie reflects his commitment to the view that Benjie, although a child, is deserving of respect. He is entitled to explanations and should have a role in decision-making. He is applying in therapeutic practice the policy recommendations now generally in effect in the context of research, which require child assent in nontherapeutic research and encourage attempts to obtain assent in therapeutic research from all children ages 7 years and older (see Chapter 13) But, why bother to do this when, as his colleague rightly points out, the outcome is a foregone conclusion, and the child is not really being given a choice? What is the point of obtaining assent, when the real consent must still come from the parents? And, could it do harm to consult the child but then not comply with his wishes?

Dr. Hartman's colleague may be questioning not only this instance of obtaining assent, but the whole trend toward greater independence for children. Would he really allow Benjie to veto a hospital stay? He wants to protect him from harm, including his own bad choices, but that can be accomplished only by restricting his liberty.

Children's Competence

This protectionist position rests on certain assumptions about children's competence. Benjie is not fully rational: he tends to see only pleasure, he is not mature enough to choose a present pain in order to achieve future benefits, and he has not had enough experience to be able to imagine what an impairment permanent hearing loss would be. The skeptical physician may have read Locke, who says that to turn a child loose to an unrestrained liberty before he has reason to guide him is to "thrust him out amongst Brutes," and Bentham who claims that the child is "too sensitive to present impulses, too negligent of the future."

The evidence about children's lack of competence can be challenged, however.

1. If one looks at decision-making as a developmental process, then one cannot treat the 18th birthday as a magic milestone at which competence and rationality spring full-born from children's heads. The 9-year-old can be expected to understand and contribute more to the process of decision-making than his 7-year-old brother, and the older teenager can contribute as an almost-adult.

2. There is some empirical evidence showing that although young children cannot give sophisticated rationales for their choices, they generally make the same treatment choices as adults (Weithorn and Campbell, 1982).

3. From a practical point of view, insofar as making decisions is a form of practical reasoning, it depends not only on cognitive capacities but to a large degree on life experience, practice in making moral judgments, and practice in disciplining oneself to act according to one's principles. Those who work with children with chronic and fatal illness find that they are much more mature in their ability to understand and make choices about their treatment than Benjie is with his very first serious ear infection.

Some people are skeptical about the value of consulting children because even if they agree to something, it is impossible to be sure that it is voluntary. This is particularly troublesome because a child is almost always in a vulnerable position toward adults. Not only are they weaker physically, for even a 10 year old can be simply carried off, but they have no power to impose their decisions on adults: all the institutions of society and access to them are controlled by adults. Even the child who needs protection from abuse from an adult needs the intervention of another adult.

There are subtle and not so subtle psychological pressures working as well. In general, children want to please their parents and may have well-hidden anxieties about being abandoned if they do not cooperate with them. The physician may be viewed as a kind friend, but even the most independent adults know that their welfare lies in the physician's hands and older children know that they need to keep the physician as a friend against the mysteries of illness and medicine. Thus, one has reason to question voluntariness even when, or perhaps especially when, assent seems to be willingly given.

A final note on voluntariness: for assent to be genuine, there must be the possibility of dissent. Children who need treatment do not really have the choice of effective dissent. Thus, their assent, one might say, is essentially meaningless. Nonetheless, there are benefits in trying to get child assent. Talking and explaining helps them to see the reasons for the medical decision and understand why they should agree. It provides a model of human relationships that are not autocratic and treats them with respect, it helps train them in decision-making, and finally, it often achieves compliance and cooperation.

Even if Benjie is not the ultimate decision-maker and does not have veto power, he can be accorded some role in decision-making. There is room for negotiation, bargaining, or even compromise. Perhaps he would settle for being able to go to MacDonald's for supper and being admitted right after that. Having a voice in deciding reinforces his sense of himself as a person and helps prepare him for the independent decision-maker he will someday be.

CHAPTER 3

Adolescent Age-Specific Values

"Out of the question! I won't wear a brace. I'll do the electrical stuff at night and anything else you want, but no brace."

"The brace is the best option for your scoliosis. Your back curvature has reached 30 degrees, and if we can't prevent it from getting to 40 degrees, it means surgery. No one wants that for you, Celia."

"But the brace is so obvious. How would you like to start high school with a big ugly brace? That's what's important to me."

How should an adolescent's values be ranked against "adult" values?

Discussion Questions

1. What are a person's "real" values and goals?
2. What weight should be given to age-specific values?

Adolescent choices are typically characterized by what might be called age-specific values, that is, values that are held only during the teen-age years or given high priority only during that time. Chief among these are concern with body image: "How do I look to others? Am I too fat, too thin, wearing the right clothes?" Also of importance is acceptance by peers and striving for independence, especially of parents.

The developmental tasks of adolescence seem to require that the individual be able to fulfill at least some of these needs. According to some psychologists, adolescents develop their own identity precisely by being concerned with their bodily image, finding a peer group that accepts them, and being able to act independently from family. Achieving these goals in adolescence paves the way for a mature and responsible adulthood.

"Real" Values and Goals

Adolescent age-specific values, however, often hold little appeal for the parents whose ultimate responsibility it is to make decisions for their child. They may see concern with body image as trivial, especially when compared with concern for good health. Even if they are sympathetic to the acute embarrassment their child would suffer from wearing a bulky back brace, they are more likely to weight long-term permanent benefits more heavily than immediate, short-term unpleasant experiences.

Age-specific values are temporary: children outgrow them and, in their own adulthood, will most likely repudiate them. So, if one were to override the adolescent's wishes, it could be justified by saying it is simply imposing the child's own later, adult values on his or her own earlier, adolescent self. Imposing a decision on another person for that person's own welfare is always a form of paternalism. As such, justification is required. Some say paternalism is justified if the person will thank you for your intervention later on. Another version of this principle is that it is justified to prevent people from choosing for themselves if they are choosing something inconsistent with their own values. Thus, if Celia's true values are those that she will have as an adult, then she should not be allowed to choose now according to her transitory adolescent values. From this it would follow that the adolescent's preference should be overridden when it conflicts with typically adult judgments of value.

It might be objected here that one cannot assume universality of adult values, which is why paternalism toward competent adults is generally not considered justified. So, why allow typical adult values to override adolescent values? If the argument is that these are the values the adolescent will later adopt, this is problematic; this adolescent may not adopt typical values.

The answer to this objection needs to be framed in practical terms. If one does not and cannot know what adult values a particular adolescent will adopt, but one does know pretty clearly that they will be different from the typical adolescent values, the best one can do is appeal to typical adult values. This is like appealing to the "reasonable person" standard: in carrying out proxy consent for those who have not had a history of well-defined values, for example for infants or severely retarded adults, one chooses for them as a reasonable person would choose.

Choosing for adolescents against their wishes assumes that their own stated preferences are not their "real" values. Of course, some adolescents do know what adult values they will adopt. Their age and behavior suggests maturity. They already have well thought-out life plans that are not transitory and that guide their choices. Unlike young children, who need protection from decisions that would preclude their having an open future, that is, the possibility of making a wide range of choices later in life, some adolescents have goals that require commitment and narrow choices. One usually does not have much of a chance of becoming a professional musician or athlete if one keeps all options open until 18 years. In such cases it seems right to let adolescents choose for themselves or, if parental consent is needed, to use the subjective standard for substituted judgment; that is, to choose as that adolescent would choose.

On the other hand, some adolescents retain their adolescent values into adulthood. To put it another way, some typically adolescent goals and values are shared by some adults. For example, successful movie stars have great concern with bodily image, no less as an adult than as an adolescent. The difference is that they retain them as adult values for good reasons, not out of developmental need.

Difficult judgments must be made by the would-be paternalist about the seriousness of an adolescent's life plan and the relation between medical choices now and the possibility of fulfilling that plan in the future. Whereas it may be irrational to allow an adolescent to refuse an appendectomy on the slight chance he may someday want to pose for the centerfold of *Playgirl* magazine, it would not be irrational to allow a high school soccer star to choose knee surgery, which carries some risk but also the promise of continued play.

Adolescent versus Adult Values

Every stage of life has its own age-specific values. Those in the prime of life may see adolescent values as trivial or shallow, but those approaching old age may regret the workaholic nature of their midlife years and criticize their own former values.

Although it is natural enough to discount adolescent values in favor of adult or prime of life values, it should not go unquestioned. One cannot argue that later is better or that values that are transitory and likely to be changed or repudiated at a later stage are to be weighted less, for then it would follow that the values of old age should be the standard by which we judge others, not prime of life values.

Adolescent values are to prime of life values as prime of life values are to old age values. We need a better justification to impose adult age-specific values on adolescents, especially when these values do not lead to choices that are irrational in the sense of being incompatible with the adolescent's own perceived life goals or so idiosyncratic that no sane adult would choose them.

One last argument against allowing children and adolescents to make decisions for themselves should be considered. It is that they suffer from lack of knowledge; that is, they do not have enough experience to be able to anticipate the future realistically; they do not know human nature well enough to know how they will feel and react in changed circumstances. This concern is well founded, but it holds, to some degree at least, against any form of advance directive. If life is a series of stages, individuals are a succession of selves, and any promise, contract, or living will one enters into binds one's future self according to present vision and values. Thus, the adolescent's decision binds her for the future in ways similar to those of more mature people. Parents and doctors may choose to keep trying to persuade Celia to accept the brace, but they should give serious consideration to her concerns, even though they may seem misguided to them.

CHAPTER 4

"Ordering Up" Medical Care

"Well, it's an unusual request. It's true that Dennis is small. He's in the 5th percentile, but we have found no metabolic abnormality. Generally growth hormone isn't prescribed unless there is abnormality. It has its dangers and I'm not sure I'd feel right giving it to Dennis."

"You don't understand, doctor. This is one very smart kid. He could go to Harvard; he could have a great career in politics, even become a Supreme Court justice. But not if he's the shortest kid in his class. Think of his self-image, think of the way others see him. It makes a difference."

"Let me look up the literature and think about this some more. Call me next week and we'll talk about it again."

How should physicians respond to requests for "designer" therapy?

Discussion Questions

1. Should physicians let parents "order up" medical care? What are the limits of such practice? When do physicians have the right to say "No"?

2. Should medicine be used for "body improvement" beyond the norm or to enhance special abilities beyond what nature has provided?

3. Should physicians ever go against their own standards to accommodate parents?

The doctor has a week of hard thinking ahead of her. Because she is being challenged by the parents' assertion of their rights as parents, she has to re-examine her role and rights as a physician. If the parents have the right to "call the shots" on certain kinds of treatment for their children, then the physician has a duty to fulfill their requests. If not, then she must find a way to explain her position and try to convince them of the unwise nature of their request. This must be done gently and firmly, if she wants to keep them as patients and have them act in their child's best interest.

The Role of Parents

What are the arguments in favor of letting parents decide? Parents have the right to choose for their children, as they see their interests. The limits of parents' freedom to choose are defined by what is illegal, seriously harmful, or defined as neglect or abuse. Within these limits, parents can impose life style, personal values, and religion pretty much as they wish. Parents can inculcate values that are materialistic or spiritual, can influence children to aim at certain goals in life, and not at others. Beyond this, parents' role is to try to provide the means to achieving their family's goals. In some cases, medicine can be the means to certain goals: this family sees the administration of growth hormone as a necessary step toward their child's achieving the goal of a successful and happy life. Given these assumptions, it seems that parents should be allowed to choose growth hormone as long as it is not illegal, seriously harmful, or defined as abuse.

In reviewing the facts about growth hormone, the physician has to concede that it is not illegal to use it and although it may carry some risk, the risk is not known to be high enough to preclude its use altogether; that is, it is prescribed for some children. Its recommended use, however, is for those with metabolic abnormality where the benefits are clearly worth the risks. If the parents were requesting something illegal, like steroids for an athletic son, or something clearly against standard medical practice, such as excessive lab tests, then obviously the physician would have no obligation to comply and indeed would have an obligation not to do so.

What makes the case of growth hormone difficult is that it is within the boundaries of good medicine, but in the doctor's judgment only barely so. What needs to be determined is whether or not the risk to the child in this case is justified by the benefit to be gained. However, who is to decide the risk/benefit ratio—physician or parents? Parents, after all, are allowed to take calculated risks for their children all the time; outside limits on what constitute acceptable risks are sometimes set by law, for example, seat belt requirements for children under age 12 years, but not everything can or should be legislated and different families have different thresholds of how much risk they can tolerate.

As part of her duty to inform, the physician certainly should provide her own best risk/benefit analysis. She might also point out that human growth hormone is a prescription drug, which suggests that professional judgment is needed; over-the-counter drugs provide parents with ultimate choice in medication. She might say, "I wouldn't prescribe it for my own child," and this may influence the parents, but Dennis is not the physician's son.

As the physician thinks about this case, she realizes that she has other reasons for not wanting to prescribe the growth hormone for Dennis. To her mind, it is a poor use of scarce resources. To some degree all prescription drugs and the time and expertise required to manufacture and administer and monitor their use are limited and expensive resources. There is some ethical requirement that would limit the use of scarce resources to their most effective therapeutic application. On the other hand, although it is unfair to those who need it more to use limited resources for less urgent reasons, the medical system in this country allows those who can pay for resources to have them. Those other children who may need it are not this physician's patients and Dennis is, and her first duty is to her own patients. Parents are not distributed fairly to those who need them most, either; Dennis is lucky to have parents who are educated enough to know about growth hormone, concerned enough to try to get it for him, and financially secure enough to be able to pay for it. They should be free to provide him with the best medical care just as they are free to provide him with the best private school education.

Conflicts about letting parents decide are, thankfully, not everyday occurrences because usually physicians and parents share the same goal, which is the good health and well-being of the child. The problem here is that the physician and the parents have different goals or, at least, see different means to the same goal and they calculate different risk/benefit ratios. The parents think the growth hormone will improve the child's life and are willing to take the risks, but the physician thinks that medicine should not be used to change normal body growth and that improvement in stature is a superficial goal. Viewed from this perspective, the problem is now not simply who should decide whether or not to give Dennis growth hormone, but who should decide Dennis' goals in life. This formulation of the issue shifts the weight toward parents' rights.

The Physician's Standards

The physician knows that some other physicians do prescribe growth hormone for normally growing children at parents' request. Part of her self-examination is to question her own standards and wonder if she should be more accommodating. Perhaps she is imposing her own personal views on this family. Since administering growth hormone is neither illegal nor absolutely against generally accepted medical judgment, perhaps her role as pediatrician does call for her to be willing to use it as the parents want. Perhaps her conscience is oversensitive and should be set aside.

The physician needs to sort out the relationship between her personal and professional values and she needs to face up to the possibility of conflict between what she personally would choose to do or would prefer to do and what she may be required to do as physician. There is a danger in trying to answer ethical questions simply by consulting one's conscience, for appeal to conscience by itself cannot justify anything (see Chapter 19). It is too subjective, too much like a personal intuition. Some of history's most vicious people claimed to have been acting from conscience, and such claims cannot be corroborated or refuted. Good intentions and good conscience are not sufficient reasons for justifying actions.

Physicians are gate-keepers; they control the use of medicine and medical techniques. The reason for this is the potential for harm; if a substance or treatment poses no potential for harm to health, then physicians should not be able to prevent its use. Thus, in the really clear cases where certain uses of medicine are illegal, harmful, or useless, physicians must say no, but they should also be able to convince parents that there are good reasons for not wanting those things for their children. Where parents are not easily convinced because what they want is not clearly illegal, harmful, or useless, perhaps physicians should re-examine their own reasons for wanting to say no.

Part I. Additional Cases for Discussion

1. A 13-year-old girl visits a health clinic to request birth control pills. Before answering any questions about herself, she asks for assurance that her parents will not be contacted.

    What should the clinic's policy be?

2. Parents request that their 6-year-old daughter be a bone marrow donor for their son with late-stage leukemia, with whom she is HLA-compatible. The girl expresses fear and resistance to the procedure.

    Should the staff comply with the parents' decision?

3. A 17-year-old male presents in the emergency room with a history of 12 hours of epigastric pain and vomiting blood and tarry stools for 2 days. Initial evaluation finds him tachycardic and mildly hypertensive, with a hemoglobin of 4.9 g/dl. Endoscopy is required to determine the site of bleeding. A blood transfusion is recommended before the procedure so that it can be performed more safely. He and his mother are practicing Jehovah's Witnesses and refuse transfusion therapy but want "everything else" done.

    Should a physician alter standards of care to comply with a patient's request?

    What options should the emergency room team pursue if agreement cannot be reached with the patient and parent?

4. A newborn with a hypoplastic left heart is stabilized with medical therapy. Surgical intervention is hazardous but offers the only possibility of sustained although limited success. The child's 17-year-old single mother adamantly refuses surgery.

    Should the medical team request a court order for surgery?

    Without surgery, should the infant be discharged to the mother's care, as she requests?

5.   A 12-year-old girl has an osteogenic sarcoma of the upper femur. The physicians recommend prompt amputation and intensive chemotherapy as the best options for cure. The parents wish to modify treatment by eliminating one drug, which has a risk of causing late-appearing heart damage. The girl, who hopes to be a dancer, appeals for a limb-salvage technique to save her leg.

Who should decide?

Part I. Suggested Reading

1. Ackerman TF. The limits of beneficience: Jehovah's Witnesses and childhood cancer. *Hastings Center Report.* 1980;10(4):13–18.
2. Gaylin W, Macklin R, eds. *Who Speaks for the Child? The Problems of Proxy Consent.* New York: Plenum Press; 1982.
3. Holder AR. Chapter V: The minor's consent to treatment. In: *Legal Issues in Pediatrics and Adolescent Medicine,* 2nd ed., New Haven: Yale University Press; 1985.
4. Jonson AR. Blood transfusions and Jehovah's Witnesses. The impact of the patient's unusual beliefs in critical care. *Crit Care Clin.* 1986;2:91–100.
5. King NMP, Cross AW. Children as decision-makers: guidelines for pediatricians. *J Pediatr.* 1989;115:10–16.
6. Lantos J, Siegler M, Cutler L. Ethical issues in growth hormone therapy. *JAMA.* 1989;461:1020–1024.
7. Leiken SL. Minor's assent or dissent to medical treatment. *J Pediatr.* 1983;102:169–176.
8. Melton GB, Koocher GP, Saks MJ, eds. *Children's Competence to Consent.* New York: Plenum Press; 1983.
9. Nazarian LF. Pediatrician's perspective. Giving to our patients—should we draw the line? *Pediatr Rev.* 1986;9:67.
10. Weithorn LA, Campbell SB. The competency of children and adolescents to make informed treatment decisions. *Child Dev.* 1982;53:1589–1598.

Part II
Telling the Truth:
What Should I Say?

CHAPTER 5

Informing Parents

"Here goes. I've hardly met these parents and I have to go and tell them their kid's been diagnosed with regional enteritis. I'll be in there all day explaining. Eleanor, you've been around here for a long time. How should I handle it?"

"Tell them everything you know and say it in simple words."

"Not very helpful, but I guess I know what you mean."

This sounds like good advice, but is not very specific. How should the resident handle the situation?

Discussion Questions

1. What is the main goal of giving parents information?
2. Can parents really understand?
3. Is it ever right to delay or withhold information?

Why Tell the Truth?

There are three quite different reasons most frequently given for requiring truth telling. Both are related to the moral and legal requirement for informed consent.

From the physicians' point of view, truth telling is a protection. This is a change from a view popular decades ago that viewed truth telling as unnecessary, a nuisance to the physician, an unwarranted burden on the patient, and a threat to the authority of the doctor-patient relationship. But time, expectations, and professional relationships have changed. The moral climate favors openness and lack of mystique, the public is more sophisticated about health and illness, and the average person welcomes the chance to participate in decision-making.

Some observers read the current moral climate pessimistically: in place of faith and confidence, patients regard practitioners with suspicion and mistrust, demand accountability, and do not hesitate to go to the courts. Expectations of what modern medicine should be able to do have risen unrealistically, while the status of physicians has fallen. In response to these changes, many physicians are beginning to see truth telling and shared decision-making as a protection for them, as a welcome relief from total responsibility for what happens to the patient. In addition, in an age of suspicion and mistrust, the physician who earns a reputation for giving clear and full information in an understandable and empathetic way builds trust, and a good doctor-patient relationship with good communication is the first defense against disaffected patients and malpractice suits.

From the patient's point of view, correct and full information is a necessity; one cannot participate in decision-making without it. Even where there are essentially no choices to be made, informed consent is required for treatment and consent cannot be informed if patients are not told or do not understand their medical situation. There is also a psychological benefit to informing people, so they can prepare themselves for whatever lies ahead. Describing the plan of treatment and the course of recovery constitutes what John Dewey calls rehearsal in the imagination, and helps both parents and child cope.

Do People Understand?

What about the skeptic's objection that patients cannot understand complicated medical information and that emotional stress reduces comprehension even more? Is there any reason other than the purely legal one to give comprehensive information?

It is true that patients often do not understand or remember what they are told. When written consent forms were first introduced, many used medical jargon or vocabulary that only college graduates could understand. Although empirical tests of later recall show that many patients do not remember what they sign, these tests do not show whether or not people understand correctly at the time they are actually signing. Those who are responsible for obtaining informed consent need to develop their own ways of knowing when the patient really is informed: by developing better consent forms and, of equal importance, by questioning, observing facial expressions, and so on. A signature at the bottom of the form may pass the legal test but does not satisfy the moral requirement.

Understanding and being informed perhaps should be viewed as a developmental process involving both cognitive powers and life experience. Parents of a child diagnosed with chronic illness or a condition requiring long-term care will grow in understanding over time and with experience. No single informing interview will ensure understanding, but the physician, nurse, and social worker have many recurring opportunities to inform and educate. Informing patients is not a one-way street. A person is not an empty receptacle that the informer fills up with facts. The process of informing is a process of communicating: giving information but also getting feedback, knowing what other people are understanding, and eliciting questions. The appropriate form for an informing interview is more like a dialogue than a lecture. Parents add both facts and values to the complete understanding of their child's medical situation and there is a richness of clinical communication when parents and physicians work together toward reasoned decision-making.

Delaying or Withholding

Another important aspect of truth telling is the question of good timing. There may be good reasons for delaying truth telling, but physicians must be sure the reasons stem from concern for the parent or child and are not their own personal reasons. It is difficult to cause pain or grief to others, and truth telling in medicine often does cause pain; but that, in itself, can never justify silence. Truth telling to parents is necessary because they must give informed consent and cannot do so without full and timely information. If the information the physician has may affect a parent's decision, then it is wrong to withhold or delay it.

There are two situations in which it is considered justified to treat a child without parental consent or to withhold the truth from parents. The first is in an emergency situation, when parents are not available to be informed and give consent. The other situation arises when the giving of information may do serious harm. The classic situation involves telling recent heart attack victims about the seriousness of their condition. Perhaps having parents in similar situations would justify not giving them all the stressful information about a child's diagnosis. However, the consequences would be compounded: there is a direct effect on parents, and indirect harm to the child who needs parental support.

Despite this possible exception to the obligation to inform parents, the physician would not be justified in making a treatment decision without consent from someone else. Since consent for a child is always proxy consent, if the parents could not be told, there would have to be an alternate named as the child's proxy and the usual rules about disclosing information would apply. Except in these special circumstances, the physician has a moral and legal duty to inform parents fully and to make every effort to be sure they both understand at the cognitive level and appreciate on the affective level. It is the mark of the skillful physician to be able to give bad news in a sensitive and empathetic way, to encourage questions and dialogue, and to have the patience to repeat information over a period of time.

CHAPTER 6

Telling the Child

"Listen to me, and pass it on to all the doctors and nurses and everyone around here: You're not to tell Franklin the name of his disease and you're not to tell him it's fatal."

"Yes, I agree with my husband. We have good reasons for asking this. First, he's so young, and 'muscular dystrophy' is a frightening name. It makes it sound so ugly. And second, you're not always right about predictions. My husband's aunt was supposed to live only a few months after they found out she had cancer, but she surprised everyone and lived for years."

Should the medical team agree?

Discussion Questions

1. What are some reasons for respecting parents' wishes? Under what conditions, if any, would someone be justified in telling the child the truth?

2. Does the fact that deception is for the child's benefit make it morally acceptable?

3. Why is it often considered justified to lie to children, but not to adults?

A great deal of latitude is generally given to parents in deciding how to raise their children, especially in their attempts to protect them from some of the harsher aspects of the grown-up world. Many parents believe that it is a young child's right to believe in Santa Claus and the tooth fairy. These beliefs seem to do no harm and may give the child a sense of security and protection. Can benevolent deception about serious illness be looked at in the same way?

Physicians usually allow parents the freedom to create whatever psychological environment they choose for their hospitalized or seriously ill child. They consider it to be the rightful realm of parents and realize that it offers a method of coping to parents who typically experience a loss of control and lose some of their sense of being able to care for and protect their child. Yet, professionals may need to draw limits, and an appropriate principle to use is one that has its origin in the Hippocratic axiom, Do no harm. So some advise respecting parents' wishes as long as they are not in conflict with good medical practice; that is, as long as they do no harm.

Reasons for Telling

Accepting this principle suggests some conditions under which it might be justified to tell the child the truth even against parents' wishes, if one has not been successful at convincing them to do so. Suppose Franklin becomes obstinate and refuses to accept treatment, objects to repeated hospitalizations, or becomes a behavior problem on the ward. Particularly if he is feeling well and experiencing few symptoms, he might say, "There's nothing wrong with me, why do I have to have all these needles, miss school, take this awful medicine?" The only way for him to make sense of his situation and be willing to comply with the treatment is by having at least some knowledge of the truth.

In the earlier days of medicine when there were no antibiotics to cure infections, and no medical methods to ensure long survival with fatal diseases such as cancer, it was easier to hide the truth from children and it probably did little harm. In the changed circumstances of modern medicine, it is more difficult to hide things and it may be more harmful.

In this case, especially in light of the prognosis of long survival, it is not clear that the parents' assumptions about the psychological effects of knowing the truth is correct. Given individual differences and the dearth of experimental data, not enough is known about how children respond. Some observers of dying children claim that children know, even without being told; they pick up cues from adults even when too young to verbalize their knowledge or questions. They experience what psychologists call "closed awareness." Also, work with children of divorcing parents suggests that the stress on the child is greater when the issues are not out in the open. Children may suspect something even worse than the reality and are deprived of the comfort and reassurance that parents can give.

A stronger principle than not doing harm is the principle that one should do whatever will benefit the child. Given the presumption in favor of parents' freedom, this principle becomes, Respect parents' wishes as long as they are in the best interest of the child. However, this is not much more than an unhelpful platitude, for controversy often arises over just that question of determining what is in the child's best interests, and the good intentions of parents or physicians cannot be simply equated with the best interest of the child.

A more helpful rule is the principle of utility, which is applied by asking, Will concealing the diagnosis, not using the name of a disease, and not speaking to the child about prognosis do more good than harm? The principle of utility allows for a more subtle analysis of the situation: one can admit that concealing the truth will likely do some harm but also will have some good effects; one needs to consider all possibilities and weigh the probable outcome. It also allows consideration of the total situation, what effects there will be on people other than the child. Are the parents so fragile that their need to control outweighs the possible harm to the child? Will conflict over truth telling destroy the doctor-parent relationship so that care of the child is compromised? Will agreeing with the parents now establish trust, so that the question can be raised again later? Will it be extremely difficult for nurses and other staff constantly to censor what they say to the child?

The problem with utilitarian reasoning is that one is always predicting consequences and one cannot be sure what will happen, but the advantage is that it is a flexible and practical way to try to decide.

Lying to Children

Why is it that we consider it justified or even required to lie to children in situations where we would think it wrong to lie to adults? One reason is that all, or almost all, lying to children is seen as benevolent deception, whereas much lying to adults is from self-serving motives. One lies to children to protect them, to prolong their innocence, to get them to do things that will benefit them, because one does not trust their judgment, because their experience is limited and they do not see dangers, because they may be tempted by unwise pleasures, or because their goals are short-term instead of long-term. On the other hand, denying children the truth always harms them to some degree by slowing their progress toward developing their own autonomy.

Letting children believe in Santa Claus may not be harmful to them, and many children and parents derive great pleasure and benefit from sharing their "false" beliefs. Some benevolent deceptions in medicine may be like this. But some can do harm, and trying to decide the balance of benefit to harm or vice versa is a helpful and morally appropriate way to decide questions of telling the truth to a child.

CHAPTER 7

When Doctors Disagree

"I think immediate amputation is needed to be sure that all the disease is removed and to guard against any possible late effects. This kind of tumor is nothing to fool around with."

"But I think we could take a 'wait and see' approach. The surgery we did got everything except a tiny portion around the vital tendons, and now if we use radiotherapy and chemotherapy together, it could be totally successful."

"What about letting Gerry's parents decide? Is that asking too much of them?"

How much should parents be told about "behind the scenes" medicine?

Discussion Questions

1. Should the parents be told about the doctors' disagreement?
2. Should the primary physician make a recommendation, or leave the choice entirely to the parents?
3. How can a recommendation be justified, in light of medical uncertainty?

Medical disagreement arises most frequently when there is genuine uncertainty about future consequences. In rapidly advancing fields such as pediatric oncology, unresolved questions are constantly under study. When the answers are in, then one can expect agreement and the treatment that works best becomes the recognized, standard treatment. But, even in more established areas of pediatrics, physicians are frequently faced with decisions about adopting a new vaccine, changing nutritional recommendations, and so on.

Telling Parents

Physicians themselves may be uneasy about dealing with medical uncertainties, and some argue that acknowledging uncertainty to parents may do harm both to the parents and to the doctor-parent relationship. Parents need to have trust and confidence in the pediatrician and that will be eroded by recognizing that even the specialists are uncertain about what to do. Further, it is an unreasonable emotional burden to impose on already stressed parents, and they cannot be expected to be able to decide for themselves when even the doctors disagree.

There are many familiar reasons for truth telling. Parents must have information in order to give legally required informed consent for treatment of their child. Parents have a moral right to make medical decisions for their own children and cannot do so without information. Withholding information, even for the most benevolent reasons, is a form of paternalism that is difficult to justify. And, to be practical, withholding information, which may or may not be a form of lying or deception, will, if discovered, result in lack of trust and resentment. Yet, the instance of uncertainty seems to present a dilemma a bit different from the usual issues about truth telling.

The Nature of Disagreements

To help answer the question about what to tell parents, physicians need to understand more clearly the nature of medical disagreements. In general, disagreements between people fall into two kinds: those about facts and those about attitudes or values. Disagreements about facts can be settled at least theoretically, if not in actual practice. If two physicians disagree about whether an X ray indicates the presence of a tumor or not, the issue can be settled by appeal to facts or data, such as an additional X ray or biopsy. For instance, if two physicians disagree about optimal treatment of a certain stage of Hodgkin's disease, the issue cannot now be settled: more information from a long-term, carefully randomized study would be required.

Medical uncertainty arises when the facts are not in. In Gerry's case, no one knows the precise likelihood of success or late effects. The evidence available does not warrant any conclusion. There is no disagreement about the facts; there is agreement that there is uncertainty. There is disagreement, however, when one physician recommends immediate amputation and the other does not. With no disagreements about the facts, the source of disagreement must be in the individual physicians' attitudes and values.

Differences in attitudes and values may be a function of one's personality and past experience—some people are conservatives and some are risk-takers—or medical training and specialty—surgeons have faith in surgery, immunologists in immunology. Once the disagreement about treatment for Gerry is recognized as disagreement in attitude or value and not about facts where the physician has expertise and can speak with authority, the question of what to tell the parents seems easier to answer. If the decision depends on being a conservative or a risk-taker, then that decision seems to be the right of the parent to make. All other things being equal, parents should be able to make decisions for their child consistent with their own values. And, of course, they cannot do this without being told that the doctors disagree and why they disagree.

Making Recommendations

Having told the parents about the uncertainty and disagreements, should physicians refrain from making any recommendations? Some would see this as an abdication of responsibility, of leaving the parents too much on their own.

What would be appropriate would be a "reasoned recommendation." Recognizing that they have resolved their own uncertainty primarily by reference to the kind of persons they are, and the values and attitudes they hold, the honest physician prefaces a recommendation with words such as these: "I prefer to be safe than sorry," "I think it's better to take a conservative approach," "As a surgeon, not doing the amputation would make me uncomfortable."

The physicians' being clear and open about their own values and reasoning helps parents to articulate their own values and reasoning. Although fully informing parents about doctors' disagreements may cause distress, nevertheless in the long run decisions made in this kind of context will be decisions parents can live with and wish to live with.

CHAPTER 8

Students, Residents, and Credibility

"Hi. I'm Faith Goodale. I am working with Dr. Creamer here in her office this month. She has asked me to see Henry and give him his weekly allergy shot. How has he been this week?"

"My, you look awfully young. Are you a real doctor? Have you ever given allergy shots before?"

How should medical students and residents present themselves to patients?

Discussion Questions

1. When is the use of the title "Doctor" appropriate, and when is it deception? If it is deception, is it ever justified?

2. How much should residents as well as medical students reveal about their status and lack of experience?

3. Do physicians owe a special duty of truth telling to their own private patients, as opposed to a clinic or emergency room population? Should concerns about credibility differ in a free clinic versus a private office?

Although the use of professional titles may seem among the more trivial of ethical dilemmas, this kind of question opens the door to examining certain aspects of the nature of the doctor-patient relationship. Even those who might tend to tell the truth without being tempted to do otherwise will profit from thinking through the reasons for truth telling, for one never knows when temptation may strike. And, assuming that deception may on occasion be justified, one needs to have some principles by which to distinguish the cases.

Against Deception

Some reasons for truth telling may be characterized as purely practical and some as purely moral. To dispense with the practical first: lying often leads to bad consequences. For self-serving reasons, if for no other, the would-be liar needs to remind herself that lying is likely to get the liar into trouble. She might be found out and if so, the damage to the personal relationship may be greater than whatever harm to oneself might have resulted from telling the truth in the first place.

Credibility in Different Settings

Since patients are in a state of relative ignorance and helplessness about medical matters, they must have trust in the good intentions of their physicians; it is an indispensable requirement in the doctor-patient relationship. Moreover, some suggest, the healer's touch can do much to enhance the therapeutic effect of drugs and other treatments, and this cannot take place without a trusting relationship. With so much at stake, is the lying worth it?

From the moral perspective, the central reason for telling the truth is respect for persons. Deception for the benefit of the deceived is a form of paternalism, and the controversy is a lively one over whether or not that is ever justified (see Chapter 1). In Faith Goodale's case, it would seem, at least on first analysis, the temptation to call herself Doctor is for her own benefit, not for the child or the mother. It would save her the trouble of explaining, save her the embarrassment of having to call in Dr. Creamer, and soothe her injured ego.

Not to tell the truth, on this analysis, would be using the other person as a means to her own end or purpose. But, as Kant insists, it is always wrong to use another person merely as a means; there is a difference between persons and things. Out of respect for the person as a rational, moral being, one has an obligation to tell the truth. The extreme instance of using persons as means is the practice of slavery, but deception, if it is not for the benefit of the deceived, is also using a person.

There are, of course, gradations of telling the truth: ways of telling not quite the truth, the whole truth, and nothing but the truth. There are a number of things Faith Goodale could say that would fall somewhere between telling the truth and deceiving. She could say, "I'm older than I look," which would evade the question, and she might get away without further explanation. Or she could evade by answering, "Well, Dr. Creamer has confidence in my ability."

As a medical student, one could not claim to be a real doctor without blatantly lying. If she were an intern, she could say, "Anyone who's graduated from medical school is a real doctor, and I do have my medical degree." This would be the truth, but maybe not the whole truth. A response that would enhance communication would be to ask the mother what she means by a "real" doctor. If she means someone with considerable experience who is practicing medicine on her own, then reference to a diploma will not do. However, if she stalls and offers the mother full answers to her questions only after the shot has been given, she would be guilty of withholding information that might have influenced the mother to act differently, for instance, asking to wait until Dr. Creamer was available.

Sometimes there is a genuine question as to what constitutes the truth. Suppose someone has never given an allergy shot before, but she has given plenty of immunizations to children. She could interpret the mother's concern as being about her deftness in giving shots, not about the particular medication. Or suppose she knows nothing about allergy shots, but Dr. Creamer has drawn up the dosage and filled the syringe for her, so her inexperience with the particular medicine is irrelevant. Would it be deception to give an answer designed to inspire confidence, or would it be just a reasonable reinterpretation of the mother's concern?

If the mother is simply looking for reassurance, is it appropriate to answer by offering just that, at the expense of an entirely truthful answer? For example, if the mother asks how much experience Faith Goodale has had, is it appropriate to answer, "Oh, I've had plenty of experience," or must she answer, "I've had six month's training on the wards at Universal hospital?" One is a factual answer, the other an evaluation, but it is her own evaluation of herself. What if six months' experience sounds like too little to the mother, but is the average training time for the kind of work she is doing; or conversely, what if it sounds alright to the mother, but she knows Dr. Creamer has started her early on independent patient care? While all of this discussion in the name of truth is going on, the poor 5-year-old, of course, is sitting nervously by, waiting to get his shot over with for another week.

Revealing Student Status

There are many other situations that raise the question of how a student doctor should present herself to parents. Often a resident, who is not a specialist in chemotherapy, acts as a "go-between" conveying information to parents. It is natural to say, "Tomorrow we are going to start high dose methotrexate," even though the resident is not part of the oncology team. The parents, because of the language, perceive her as competent to make medical judgments, not as a mere go-between. Is this deception? It soothes the parents to think they are talking with someone who really knows, but the resident must be nervous: one more question and she will have to admit that she knows only what she has been told.

A similar question about deception arises when a student doctor approaches a patient to do a procedure for the first time. Although one could say that patients who come to a teaching hospital acknowledge and accept the fact that they will be treated by doctors-in-training—indeed, proper admission and consent forms should say this—parents expect that the doctor who treats their child is there primarily as therapist, not as student. Yet, for each student doctor there must be a first time and a first patient.

Again, Kant's principle that it is wrong to treat people merely as means is helpful. Is the student poking and probing repeatedly, just for her own benefit? Is the imposition on the child relatively harmless or does it pose a risk? Should a student's first spinal tap be done on a suspected intracranial bleed, where a tap that accidentally nicks a blood vessel will ruin the diagnostic value of the sample, or in a less urgent clinical situation?

The question of who counts as a "real" doctor may be relative, even within our own culture. Although the legal requirements for practicing medicine are set by state boards of health, in actuality the amount of training and experience required to perform specific medical procedures may vary with the setting. In rural areas where doctors are scarce and specialists nonexistent, the same physician may be encouraged by the hospitals and the respective communities to function as anesthesiologist, surgeon, obstetrician, and medical examiner, despite only modest training in any of these special areas. In an impoverished city hospital, house staff are allowed, or required, to do many things they would not be asked or permitted to do in a better staffed institution. To a clinic patient with no choice about physicians, anyone who offers medical help is probably going to be accepted gratefully as a real doctor.

Medical students or residents might resent having their credibility questioned in the clinic setting, as opposed to the private pediatrician's office. Yet, if one respects the Kantian principle that truth is due a person simply out of respect for one's status as a person, the setting should be irrelevant and all patients should be invited into a doctor-patient relationship based on truthfulness and trust. The practical circumstances may be different—the clinic doctors rotate and there is less risk of deception being found out—but the moral basis for truth telling remains the same.

Part II. Additional Cases for Discussion

1. A nurse caring for a child on a treatment protocol notices that one drug was inadvertently omitted in the past. Although not likely to affect the outcome, she wonders if the parents should be told.

    How should errors in care be handled?

2. A 14-year-old boy with sickle cell disease has been having frequent pain crises requiring hospitalization. Each attack has lasted more than a week and responded only to parenteral narcotics. Based on hemoglobin S levels and stressful social events at the time of the attacks, there is concern that his pain may not have an organic basis. Because of the fear of narcotic addiction, several nurses and residents propose giving the patient a placebo.

    When, if ever, might use of a placebo be justified?

3. A 12-year-old girl recently admitted to the hospital is found to have a widely invasive brain tumor. Her parents, on learning that she has only a short time to live, ask various members of the staff what to tell their daughter.

    What should be considered in deciding whether or not to tell the truth?

    Should it make a difference if the child is likely to survive days, or months, or a year?

4. Parents have just been informed that their son has cancer. The distraught mother appeals to the physician, "Tell me he'll make it!" The father asks, "What's going to happen now?"

    How much of the whole truth is required and when?

Part II. Suggested Reading

1. Basson MD, Dworkin G, Cassell EJ. The "student doctor" and a wary patient. *Hastings Center Report.* 1982;12(1):27–28.
2. Bluebond-Langner M. *The Private Worlds of Dying Children.* Princeton, NJ, Princeton University Press; 1978.
3. Bok S. Lying to children. *Hastings Center Report.* 1978:8(3):10–13
4. Brody H. The lie that heals: the ethics of giving placebos. *Ann Intern Med.* 1982;97:112–118.
5. Hirshuat Y, Bleich D. Choosing a therapy when doctors disagree. *Hastings Center Report.* 1975;5(2):19–20.
6. Katz J. Why doctors don't disclose uncertainty. *Hastings Center Report.* 1984;14(2):35–44.
7. Ladd RE, Forman EN. Telling the truth in the face of medical uncertainty and disagreement. *Am J Pediatr Hematol Oncol.* 1989;11(4):463–466.

Part III
Deciding Not to Treat:
What Are the Limits?

CHAPTER 9

Impaired Newborns

"Let's begin morning rounds. Baby H was born at a gestational age of 26 weeks and weighed 590 grams. His eyelids were partially fused and at 1 minute the Apgar score was 1 with no spontaneous respirations, but a slow heartbeat was detected. The baby was resuscitated and put on a respirator. After 24 hours he had severe respiratory distress syndrome and ultrasound revealed a grade IV intraventricular hemorrhage. Aggressive respiratory support now will somewhat increase the baby's chances of survival, but even if he does survive, he will likely have significant brain damage and pulmonary dependency. Any questions?"

"Yes, I have a basic problem with this case. Do we, as hospital staff, have to keep supporting this infant? Isn't it hopeless and even cruel? Has anyone discussed this with the parents?"

When, if ever, is withdrawal of life support from infants permissible, legally and morally?

Discussion Questions

1. What are the federal and American Academy of Pediatrics (AAP) guidelines on treatment of impaired newborns?

2. Is there a moral difference between deciding not to initiate treatment at birth and deciding to withdraw treatment later?

3. What are some further questions not addressed by the guidelines?

The joy of parents whose premature baby is saved by modern medical technology is enormous. Yet, the use of the same kind of technology to sustain the life of those newborns whose conditions are incompatible with continued life or who are so severely impaired that they are not conscious of life raises a great number of intellectually perplexing and emotionally charged ethical dilemmas.

These are the issues that probably cause the greatest degree of agony and the largest number of disagreements between physicians, between medical staff and parents, and among those theorists who try to conceptualize the issues.

One positive outcome of the otherwise unfortunate federal attempts at regulating hospital practice by the so-called Baby Doe regulations is the attention given to these issues by both public and medical groups. Attempts to set forth guidelines by the AAP and others have gone a long way toward clarifying the issues, although certainly not achieving unanimity of opinion.

Guidelines and Their Weaknesses

All those charged with the care of newborns need to be clear on the legal and ethical status of the various guidelines and their implications. Briefly stated, recommended guidelines include the duty to treat in emergency or doubtful situations, the absence of obligation to pursue clearly futile treatment, and the acceptability of withholding treatment under certain specified conditions. Pediatricians will need to consult state laws to see if there are more specific mandates or restrictions.

1. In emergency situations, treat. An emergency situation is defined as one that is unanticipated and life threatening or where lack of immediate treatment will increase risk to health or where treatment is needed to alleviate physical pain or discomfort. With newborns in distress, time is important; when there has been no opportunity to assess the infant's condition and immediate resuscitation will sustain life, the accepted policy is to treat now and ask questions later.

In general, neonatal intensive care unit (NICU) policy is posited on a presumption in favor of treating infants. The burden of proof is on the proponent of not treating. This policy seems justified by the increasingly good outcomes for those preemies who need temporary help at the time of birth and by the increasing capacity of surgery to correct what used to be lethal deformities. Moreover, the chance that delay in treating may result in losing an infant with an otherwise good prognosis overrides the possibility that the team may sustain an infant who, on closer examination, it may have been morally justified not to try to save.

An advantage of viewing the immediate treatment of newborns as emergency treatment is that emergency treatment, even for an older child, is always acceptable, even without parental consent. This is because of the reasonable assumption that it is what people would want. In addition, for newborns, blanket consent for needed medical treatment usually has already been given in the mother's consent form for admission for labor and delivery.

Immediate treatment can buy time to clarify diagnosis and prognosis, and to inform and consult with parents. The reasonableness of such a policy, however, depends on the willingness to defer, not rule out, decisions about nontreatment.

Initiating versus Withdrawing Treatment

It used to be thought that initiating treatment meant a commitment to continued treatment. One result was that physicians were sometimes too cautious about using artificial life support. Recognizing that whatever conditions might support a decision not to initiate treatment should also support a decision to withdraw treatment, then the use of initial treatment as a temporizing measure makes good sense and is good medical practice.

When it comes to refraining from initiating treatment versus withdrawing treatment, the psychological difference is admittedly very real, but the moral difference is not. If there are good moral reasons for not initiating treatment, and the same reasons still hold a bit later for withdrawing treatment, then withdrawing is not any more wrong than not initiating would have been.

2. Clearly futile treatment is not morally required. According to the guidelines developed by the AAP in conjunction with other advocate groups, if medical care is clearly beneficial, then the infant should always be treated, but if treatment will be clearly futile or will only prolong dying, it is justified to withhold it. Although the AAP does not define futile treatment, it is clear that what is meant is treatment that is futile in terms of the infant's survival.

The life of the infant is further protected in these guidelines by the stipulation that the medical condition of the infant should be the sole criterion for withholding treatment, that is, not the wishes of the parent or the cost to others. This seems to mean, for example, if the infant is under a certain weight, where there is no known survival of infants that small—or no known survival under the best conditions this particular hospital and staff can offer, and transport is not available—then resuscitation and life support efforts need not be undertaken.

Treatment is also futile if the infant has some physical impairment incompatible with life which is uncorrectable, for example, certain cardiac malformation or lack of sufficient intestines. If this is apparent at birth, no treatment need be initiated. If it becomes known only later, then no further treatment need be initiated at that point.

3. If treatment is not medically indicated, there is no moral obligation to treat. According to the proposed federal regulations of December 1985, struck down by the Supreme Court in 1986 but incorporated into policy in some states, treatment is not medically indicated if the physician, according to reasonable medical judgment, determines that any of these conditions exists:

1.   the infant is chronically and irreversibly comatose,
2.   treatment would merely prolong dying,
3.   treatment would not be effective in correcting all of the life-threatening conditions,
4.   treatment would be futile in terms of physical survival,
5.   treatment would be virtually futile and inhumane.

Many pediatricians find these guidelines ambiguous and open to interpretation. One reasonable interpretation is that in general there is no obligation to treat on the remote chance of success, especially when the treatment would produce severe and prolonged suffering.

Judging whether or not a treatment is inhumane raises questions about whether or not newborns feel pain, whether physical pain and mental suffering of infants can be distinguished as they are for adults, and what are the "tolerable limits" of pain for newborns. It used to be general practice to do surgery on newborns without anesthetic, and it has been shown that children are generally given pain medication up to one quarter less than the relative amount administered to adults with the same surgery. New information about infants' pain perception requires that these practices be re-examined.

4. Medically indicated treatment may not be withheld. This kind of treatment is defined as whatever is likely to be effective in ameliorating or correcting all life-threatening conditions. The bottom line here clearly is sheer survival. The implication is that treatment may not be withheld based on judgments about quality of life.

The life of the infant is protected in the AAP guidelines by stipulating that if it is uncertain that medical care will be beneficial, treatment is not necessarily required, but if it is withheld, then the infant's disability should not be the basis of withholding treatment. If in doubt at any point, the presumption is in favor of treating. They further hold that if medical care is clearly beneficial, that is, in terms of survival, then treatment is required and the medical condition of the infant should be the sole criterion, presumably ruling out wishes of the parents, cost, and so forth.

These guidelines appear to be quite specific and capture a consensus of what constitutes good medical practice and they should have the effect of standardizing practice across the country. However, according to a 1986 survey of neonatologists, a significant number judged that in the several cases used as samples, maximal life-prolonging treatment would not be in the best interests of the infant described, for example, a full-term infant with trisomy 13 who develops congestive heart failure at 3 weeks of age, even though the federal "Baby Doe" regulations would require it. Also, a large percent of the respondents believe that the regulations interfere with parents' rights to decide what is in their children's best interests and that the regulations do not allow adequate consideration of the infants' suffering.

5. In cases of disagreements or uncertainty about whether or not treatment is required, an Infant Care Review Committee/Ethics Committee may be consulted. There are cases that do not clearly meet the guidelines, and many hospitals have set up special committees to help resolve these situations.

Further Questions

In addition to these published and generally accepted guidelines, there are a number of questions, the answers to which rest on contested principles, still very much under debate.

1. May treatment be withheld if parents request it? Surely no—if it clearly benefits the child. Surely yes, if it clearly meets the conditions set down in the proposed federal regulations, cited above.

On the other hand, if the usefulness of the treatment is uncertain or ambiguous, or if several physicians disagree about whether or not treatment is medically indicated, then it seems reasonable to defer to parents' wishes. However, it should be noted that it is always possible under federal and/or state regulations for someone to make allegations against a physician and/or hospital for suspected medical neglect.

In unambiguous cases, if parents refuse consent for life-saving therapy and in the physicians' reasonable medical judgment the child will not be chronically and irreversibly comatose, the treatment will be effective in correcting all life-threatening conditions, will not merely prolong dying, will not be futile in terms of survival, and will not be virtually futile and inhumane, then physicians may have to request a court order for treatment.

A separate issue is this: Should treatment be continued when parents request it, even if medical staff consider it futile? Consideration must be given to factors such as misunderstanding, denial, religious beliefs, and psychological needs of the parents, but also to use and misuse of professionals' time, medical resources, and the psychological impact on staff asked to do what they know is futile. Some are now arguing that in certain circumstances it would be morally wrong to accede to parents' wishes to treat (see Chapter 19).

2. May nontreatment decisions be based on quality of life? Those who support the idea specify it in different ways. The President's Commission on medical ethics suggests that treatment may be withheld when handicaps are so severe that continued existence would not be a net benefit to the infant. This is a strict criterion in that only the benefits and burdens on the infant are considered, not those on parents or society.

The quality of the child's life also depends on the willingness and ability of the family to provide support and care. Some social critics would also consider the role of the community; unless society can offer handicapped individuals appropriate homes and rehabilitative services to assure a good quality of life, federal regulations should not mandate treatment, especially against parental wishes.

3. May futile treatment be continued for purposes of future knowledge? In pushing the boundaries of better care for premature and impaired infants, the boundaries between treatment and research become more blurred. It is always a relevant question to ask: Why are we doing this? Do we really think it will help the baby or are we hoping to find out something? Nontherapeutic research on children is never morally required and parents should always be given the chance to refuse procedures that are not expected to benefit their child (see Chapter 13).

4. Are food, water, and palliative care always required? The same debate about withholding food and water from dying persons applies to children as well as adults. Courts have found that nutrition and hydration in any form may be considered medical treatment, depending on the clinical circumstances. Thus,

they may be withdrawn under the same guidelines as other treatment. At the heart of the matter is that the child not be made to suffer needlessly.

5. Are cost and use of resources relevant factors in nontreatment decisions? With increasing national concern about escalating medical costs, this question cannot be ignored. It often arises when one must make room in an already crowded NICU for yet another infant.

Although no one wants to set a value on life or an upper limit on expenditures for life-sustaining treatment, if treatment is virtually futile, there may be pressure to have parents agree to withdrawal, and when prognosis for a minimally good quality of life is very poor, even if the child does not appear to be suffering, there may be sentiment to end treatment.

Babies whose lives have been saved but cannot live outside a hospital environment create strains of enormous proportions on hospital staff and public or private insurance funds. Yet, to advocate nontreatment for these children may go well beyond considerations of the benefits and burdens of continued existence to the infant, and must be approached with caution.

CHAPTER 10

Considering Quality of Life

"Doctor, you look surprised that I'm asking if Inez's respirator can be turned off. Look, what kind of life does she have? She's 5 years old and has been in the hospital most of the time. She can't eat normally, and because of the dysfunctional bowel problem, even tube feedings don't work. So, she needs a central line, and it keeps coming out and has to be replaced surgically. She can't breathe properly, so she has that tracheostomy, which needs aspiration several times a day, and she struggles against that. Even though her mental age is only 2 or 3 months, I know she feels things. Sometimes I think I see her smile a little bit, but most of the time I think she's feeling pain."

"You're right. It would be easier if she had no consciousness at all, for example, if she were in a persistent vegetative state."

"But she is conscious, and her life is so poor, so minimal. I've heard that sometimes other parents like me decide enough is enough. Shouldn't we be thinking of something like that?"

Should quality of life ever be a decisive reason for withdrawing life-support therapy?

Discussion Questions

1. What are the arguments against considering quality of life in nontreatment decisions? Can these arguments be answered?

2. Is all life, any life, valuable? Equally valuable?

3. What might be a reasonable criterion for quality of life decisions?

The successes of medicine present us with some of its most agonizing ethical dilemmas. With meticulous nursing care, Inez will continue to live. But are the occasional pleasurable feelings that make her smile enough to make life worth living to her? How can her moments of discomfort be weighed into the balance? And how dare someone else make that determination for her?

There are three situations where nontreatment is generally accepted.

1. There is brain death. Even though heart-lung function can be sustained artificially, where there is no brain function, there is no life and that is the end of treatment.

2. The child is in a persistent vegetative state and there is virtually no hope of recovery. There is little if any controversy that it is not required, legally and morally, to sustain life functions for such a child.

Inez does not fit into either of these categories; she has brain function and some affective responses. Yet, she is barely above being in a vegetative state.

3. Treatment is clearly futile. Unfortunately, there is an ambiguity in the term "futile" that can lead to miscommunication. One physician may mean that no treatment will recover the child's lost functions or improve her condition. Another reserves judgments of futility to apply only to children who are dying and cannot survive. One must ask, "futile relative to what?" It will be easier to justify non-treatment when survival is unlikely than when treatment is futile relative to improved status.

Since Inez is neither brain dead, nor in a persistent vegetative state, nor unlikely to continue to survive with proper care, any question about not continuing treatment will have to be based on quality of life. To say that this is a controversial area is to understate the issue.

Arguments Against Quality of Life

The arguments against any consideration of quality of life has a long, proud history. Human life is of unqualified value, it is said. To judge one life worth living and another not is to deny the essential equality of all people, to discriminate against some, and to devalue what is sacred. To judge with the purpose of denying life to some would be to arrogate power that should be only God's.

These views, whether in a religious or secular form, are ingrained in the Western religious and democratic traditions and cannot be ignored. As commonly invoked, however, they can be shown to be confused and inconsistent with other commonly held beliefs about the value of life. There are a number of claims that need to be considered.

1. "Judging quality of life implies valuing some lives more than others, and this is morally wrong because all human life is equally valuable."

Notice the equating of "valuing lives" to "the value of life." What it implies is that sheer life in the most fundamental biological sense is to be valued. If so, then we should sustain all human organisms or even parts of organic systems in any way possible.

If, on the other hand, it is human lives that are valued, then that is a different story. Human lives are biographical lives—persons with a history, some consciousness, some pleasures, desires, or interests, perhaps memory, and those with potential for these things—and the class of biographical lives is considerably smaller than the class of biological human life.

On the basis of this crucial difference, a meaningful quality of life distinction can be drawn. Those biological human beings who have lives or potential for lives have high or unconditional value, whereas those that are biologically alive but have no potential for lives in the sense defined have lower or conditional value. So one confusion is clarified. Whereas one would not want to say that biological life has no value at all, its real value is instrumental in that it allows one to have a biographical life.

Furthermore, of those who have human lives, it is hard to deny that different lives are considered of different value, that is, more desired or sought after. It just is not true that all human lives are held to be of equal value. Quality of life decisions recognize the fact that some kinds or qualities of life are more desired and some are ranked so low as not to be desired at all. Inez's future may well fall into this category.

2. "Judging quality of life in the context of refusing treatment implies that not all life is good and that sometimes death may be better than life. But that is not true. Life is always good and death is always bad by comparison. A rational person would always choose life over death."

For Socrates, there are moral limits, for others, physical limits where living is worse than dying. Once that has been granted, then the life–death, good–bad identification has been abandoned and the way is open to judge some ways of living life as good or better and some as not so good, to the point that death may be preferable. One could even go on to say that if death is better than a given way of living, then it would be wrong to require life.

3. The slippery slope argument: "If we allow refusal of treatment for those who are just above a vegetative state, it will be easier to begin to allow refusal at less severe stages, even to those just barely below normal functioning, and to move or slip from the wholly voluntary to the completely involuntary."

There will always be difficult borderline cases, of course, but one cannot refuse to make any distinction among cases in a desperate effort to avoid either misapplication to inappropriate cases or a gradual weakening of the criterion to apply to too many cases. As Sartre said in a slightly different context: Not to choose is to choose. So, to refuse to use a quality of life criterion for even quite clear cases does not avoid making a moral judgment; it just makes a moral judgment that is untenable.

A Reasonable Criterion

What can now be said in favor of quality of life decisions? A strong argument would be that some lives are so unbearable that to continue them is wrong in itself. A less emotional argument would be a utilitarian one: weighing benefits and burdens. Considering only the benefits and burdens to the child herself, one asks: Do the moments of pleasure that Inez has outweigh the unpleasant moments—in frequency, duration, intensity? The ratio is one that changes as her physical condition changes and the various procedures required to sustain her life. If suctioning is required more frequently, if episodes of surgical intervention increase, then the burdens begin to outweigh the benefits.

Benefits and burdens to another are always difficult to measure, but in practical terms a judgment can often be made that will be acknowledged by staff and family alike. And when that happens, stopping treatment may be seen to be in the best interest of the child.

CHAPTER 11

"Do Not Resuscitate"

"Oh, doctor! Help her, save her! She can't breathe. She's going to die. It's never been this bad before."

"Okay, okay. Let's go over here and talk for a second. The ER people will make her comfortable. We've been dealing with Janine's cystic fibrosis for a long time now. Remember—we all knew this was coming, and you and Janine and I talked about it several times and she said she didn't want to go through resuscitation again, didn't want to end up on a respirator for months before she died. She's 17 now and very mature, and we all agreed to go along with her wishes. You signed the DNR for her, saying comfort measures only. Are you sure you want to go back on that now?"

What are the medical staff's obligations concerning do not resuscitate (DNR) orders for children?

Discussion Questions:

1. Is there an obligation to discuss options about resuscitation measures?

2. Is deciding to limit resuscitation measures morally different from other nontreatment decisions?

3. What are the problems with advance directives?

We can do it, but should we? This is one of the most frequently asked questions in medical ethics today. Resuscitative measures are among the miracles of modern medicine. They can stave off death until the body returns to independent functioning or they can be used repeatedly or continuously to keep bodily systems functioning virtually endlessly.

Hospital DNR policies represent one of the most forthright and thoughtful steps that organized medicine has taken to address the ethical issues posed by the increased capabilities of medical technology. In keeping with common moral feelings, the presumption is that total support will be given to all patients unless there are special instructions to the contrary. Written orders can specify which measures are to be given and which to forego. The orders are documented in the chart, made known to all personnel caring for the patient, and reviewed and updated at frequent intervals. Since different levels of resuscitative measures may be specified, the preference is to speak of Orders about Resuscitation Measures (ORM) instead of DNRs. The orders reflect discussion and agreement

between physicians and the competent adult patient or the proxies for an
incompetent patient.

The Physician's Obligation

The ORM option is considered a positive thing by those who choose it. Although
in many instances resuscitative measures are a definite benefit to the patient,
they can be physically painful and psychologically traumatic. Therefore, the
usual calculation of benefit and burdens is relevant, acknowledging that in some
cases the benefit will not outweigh the burdens.

Thus, if one grants that having ORM options can be a good thing and that
there are reasonable grounds for an adult to choose it, not making it available for
children or not presenting it as an option to a particular family whose child
would meet the hospital guidelines would be withholding something desirable
from them, penalizing children for being minors who cannot make choices for
themselves.

Physicians in general are not aggressive about using ORM options. The
question is why not. Do they avoid it to protect themselves from having to think
about it or from difficult discussions with patients, or do they do it to protect the
patients? If the latter, then one must question again the pattern of paternalism
(see Chapter 1) that characterizes many aspects of many doctor–patient
relationships.

The "old way" of dealing with difficult questions such as death and dying is
by what psychologists call closed awareness. The doctor knows the patient is
dying, the patient (even a young child) and the family know, and they know that
the others know but they do not talk about it. It makes everything easier for both
parties in that there are no painful conversations, no painful decisions, and the
course of events is inevitable. On the other hand, if there are real choices to be
made, it is the family and not the physician who should make them, and
paternalistic attitudes do not allow this. The family is harmed by not being able
to choose for their child according to their own preferences and values, and the
child may be harmed by not having ORM available when it would be a benefit to
her. Thus, in the interests of family autonomy, truth telling, antipaternalism, and
the best interest of the child, the physician does have the obligation to discuss
ORM when the child's condition warrants it.

ORM versus Other Nontreatment Decisions

Limiting resuscitative measures and withdrawing life supports, like withdrawing
ventilator support or withholding antibiotics, are ways of foregoing treatment.
The perceived difference is that ORM is an omission of something that might be
done, whereas disconnecting a respirator or feeding tube is an act of

commission. It has been argued here that while there may be a psychological difference, there is no significant moral difference. If foregoing treatment is a reasonable decision, and the decision is made with attention to informed consent, how or when it is accomplished is not a moral sticking point.

However, there are some features of ORM that are of moral interest. Because it is an open issue and has been openly debated in the public arena, and because there is moral consensus to the extent that a hospital policy is written and made public, it has a greater moral force than other, more private decisions. A family can measure its own situation and reasons against criteria found reasonable by others and may feel more confirmed in their judgment that it is an accepted and humane way to approach the death of a suffering child. The psychological advantage of ORM is that the time of its implementation is set by natural events. The implementation of a decision to withdraw ventilator support can drag on indefinitely; the family may agree in principle but have a hard time deciding that now is the time. Once ORM has been decided, it is out of anyone's hands when the final failure of the bodily systems will come.

Problems with Advance Directives

ORM, living wills, and durable powers of attorney are all referred to as advance directives. Since the parents or guardians are legally designated proxies for their children, and since they are competent and generally available to give consent when decisions arise, living wills and durable powers of attorney are not applicable. Situations calling for resuscitative measures, however, may arise when parents are not immediately available, so ORM is as relevant for children as for adults.

There are two important problems that must be faced.

1. Discussion about ORM can be very stressful for families (and for older children and teens who take part in their own medical decisions) and it may do harm even to bring it up. They will interpret it to mean that their child is dying, which is correct, and that death is imminent, which may not be correct, and that the doctor knows something that he or she is not telling them, which is incorrect.

The solution to this problem is not to refrain from the discussion but to think carefully about the manner of presentation. The goal is to be open, honest, and informative so parents can consider and decide. Further, the goal is to minimize anxiety and to frame the discussion so parents are always able to keep hope alive. Families can be realistic and still hopeful.

There is room for physician discretion about initiating discussion of ORM. If there is good evidence that such a discussion will not only be stressful but unduly stressful or do serious harm to particularly fragile parents, the obligation to discuss may be overridden. In such cases, especially with competent adults, it is suggested that the physician use general language and try to elicit general preferences about vigorous methods of sustaining life. This seems insufficient for writing ORM.

2. What happens if people change their mind after agreeing to ORM? As noted before, almost always the presumption is in favor of total support. Thus, if there is any question about the validity of ORM, most care-givers will resuscitate first and ask questions later. In the case of living wills and durable powers of attorney, any orders not to treat may be rescinded at any time, just by verbal request and even, for some policies, by incompetent patients.

Families like Janine's who have carefully and thoughtfully arranged for ORM may panic at the last minute. If they are with the child when cardiac arrest occurs or when she is struggling for breath, even though orders for no ventilator support have been given, they may well give verbal directions against the ORM. It will be a very difficult task for the attending physician and nurse to determine whether the parents have really had a change of heart and regret the earlier decision or whether their present objection comes about as a reflex reaction at the time of stress. If the latter seems the more likely and if time permits, the care-givers can gently remind the family of their earlier decision, point out that the child's suffering will be prolonged by resuscitation, and then see how the family responds.

CHAPTER 12

Hastening Death

"Katie's suffering is so awful. We're her parents and we've been here all day long and we know what she's going through."

"Yes, neuroblastoma with bony metastases is really bad. We're trying our best to control the pain."

"This can't go on. There's no point to it. I wouldn't let my dog die like this. Can't you do something to get it over with more quickly?"

Is active euthanasia ever morally justified?

Discussion Questions

1. Would active euthanasia be incompatible with the role of the physician and nurse, or with the goals of medicine?

2. What is the moral difference, if any, between withdrawal of treatment, giving DNR orders, administering a massive dose of morphine, or a lethal dose of potassium chloride?

3. If active euthanasia were morally acceptable, what role should physicians play?

However many times a physician, nurse, or social worker shares with a family the dying of their child, the agony of it and the sense of helplessness is renewed. Yet, if parents appeal for help in enabling the child to die more quickly and less painfully, this presents a tremendous conflict for the professional. There is compassion for the family and child but there is also a professional commitment to preserving life.

Goals of Medicine

The goals of medicine are multiple, however, and besides the duty to preserve life and to do no harm, there is also a duty to reduce suffering when possible. How can these goals be reconciled in the face of an appeal for active euthanasia?

Traditionally, a strong argument has been made against active euthanasia by trying to draw a clear distinction between killing and letting die. Killing is an active intervention that results in death for a person who would not otherwise die or who would not die at that time. Letting die is a passive standing back, letting nature take its course. The argument is that killing is morally wrong, but since letting die is not the same as killing—one does not do anything to cause death, one does not intend death, and death is not certain—then letting die can be morally acceptable. Many decisions not to initiate treatment or to withdraw treatment from dying patients are justified in this way.

However popular this argument, the distinction between the active and the passive is dubious, for often the intent and the consequence of both are identical. The would-be murderer who is lucky enough to find his intended victim drowning in a pond and does nothing to save him is as morally responsible for the death as if he had thrown him into the water: he intended him to die and he did die, in the one case because of something the murderer did and in the other case because of something he purposely failed to do.

In the case of modern medicine, it is hardly ever really fair to say that we are "letting nature take its course." Furthermore, although most often medical intervention helps the patient, when it fails it can bring on a greater degree of suffering than if there had been no medical intervention at all. It used to be said that pneumonia was "the old man's friend," but almost never is anyone allowed to die of pneumonia any more: the pneumonia, which would have resulted in a peaceful, comparatively easy death, is treated and the patient lives on, only to die a bit later with prolonged and greater discomfort.

Given this understanding of the intervention of medicine and the criticisms of the moral significance of the active–passive distinction, a new argument could be made: there is no real moral difference between killing and letting die, so if letting die is sometimes morally acceptable, then killing may be sometimes acceptable. Since one of the goals of medicine is to reduce suffering, and since some forms of dying involve great suffering, it may be acceptable in some cases to use medicine to hasten death or to produce a less difficult dying. In other words, it is not necessarily incompatible with the professional duties of the doctor to become involved in active euthanasia.

Moral Differences

It must be remembered that killing is illegal and fatal injections will be interpreted by a jury as homicide. What counts as murder or homicide in both morality and law takes into account motivation, and a position based on the philosophical principle of double effect has been adopted by the American Medical Association and many other health-care professionals.

The principle of double effect makes the morality of an act depend on its intent, not its consequences. It says it is permissible to do something, knowing it will result in something bad, if it is intended to bring about something good and it is the only way to bring about the good. You may not do something bad in order to bring about something good, but you may do something knowing it will have both a good and a bad effect. Applied to medicine, then, physicians may administer large amounts of morphine with the intention of alleviating suffering, even though they know that the morphine will depress respiration and may bring about a quicker death. This is acceptable, whereas an injection of potassium chloride, which can have as its direct intent only to bring about immediate death, is not permissible.

To many, this seems like a distinction without a difference. The emphasis on intention is appropriate, but why not be honest and say outright that it does seem justified to hasten death in some cases? There is, after all, a big difference between causing death with the intent of relieving suffering and causing death in order, say, to get someone's money.

A conservative approach might be to say this: active euthanasia may be considered if and only if the child is dying, the condition causing death cannot be medically reversed, and the benefits of living are exceeded by the child's suffering, that is, there is conscious suffering, and the point has been reached where increased pain medication will either lead directly to death or will result in the child being "doped" into nearly continuous unconsciousness. In other words, active euthanasia would be morally acceptable only for someone who is dying, with no way to preserve life, and as a measure to prevent suffering.

The Role of the Physician

A further question concerns the role of the physician. Even if active euthanasia or assisting in a suicide became morally accepted, should the physician be involved? Many fear that if the physician has a dual role, both as healer and as agent of death, the trusting relationship so important between patient and physician would be destroyed.

There are two kinds of answers to this objection. The first one assumes that it is always bad to die. When one begins to envision situations where continued life is more of a burden and the death is a release from suffering, the physician is seen not as executioner, but as savior from suffering and the only one available to play this role. The second answer has to do with the worry that a physician might decide to end a child's life while the parents still want to keep fighting for life. This concern can be resolved by making sure that the physician is not the sole decision-maker. A mechanism must be developed, perhaps a special committee, and with careful attention to the informed consent of the family or guardian.

Other concerns include guilt of the parents and the possibility of error in prognosis. Both of these concerns can be addressed by comparing the decision to withdraw or not initiate further aggressive treatment, that is, passive measures, with the proposed active measures. There is always the possibility of error, but no more in the one case than in the other. A further concern is that active euthanasia guarantees death, but passive withdrawal leaves open the possibility of not dying. There is always the possibility of regret or guilt on the part of parents, but usually much less so with those who have had time to think it through and are convinced, intellectually and emotionally, that they are doing the right thing for their child and who have the support of their medical caregivers.

The larger question is this: when death is inevitable, should people be able to have some control over the time and manner of their death? The religious answer is often an unequivocal no; life and death are in the hands of God and humans should not interfere. The underlying theme is hidden by rhetoric about the sanctity of human life. Is it really honoring life by allowing people to die in unnecessary pain? Or, is it a side-stepping of the duty to relieve pain to say one should not interfere?

The climate of opinion about medicine and death and dying is changing. The Netherlands has recently enacted legislation permitting voluntary, physician-assisted suicide or active euthanasia. It is an idea whose time may be coming. There is, as always though, a special problem about children. Since they cannot choose and consent for themselves, there can be no such thing as voluntary euthanasia for children. On the other hand, should children be "punished" by the fact that they are children and cannot choose it for themselves? Future generations may look back at us today and wonder how we could have been so barbaric as to allow children to die under the conditions described in this case.

Part III. Additional Cases for Discussion

1. A 7-year-old girl has been in a persistent vegetative state since being hit by a car 6 months ago. Although not requiring a respirator, she is dependent on nasogastric feedings. Her father now requests that the feeding tube be removed. One house officer, concerned about the child "drying up" over days, asks, "If you're going to pull the tube, why not end it quickly with morphine?"

    Is there a moral and/or legal difference between
    1. pulling the plug of a respirator
    2. discontinuing tube feedings
    3. giving a lethal dose of morphine?

    Would removing the tube be killing the child or letting her die? Is there a moral difference?

2. A 1-year-old child with a brain tumor will die in a few months without intensive therapy. With treatment, 50% will still succumb, and among the survivors, only one in four will have an IQ greater than 80. The parents refuse therapy.

    How should the physician respond?

    What if two-thirds of the survivors were likely to have normal intelligence?

3. A newborn is found to have a short-gut syndrome. Despite being told that parenteral nutrition will be required indefinitely to sustain life and even so, that the child is likely to die within a few years, the parents plead for such treatment.

    Should physicians comply with the parents' request?

    Should this be a decision for the family and physician alone?

4. A 12-year-old boy with progressive renal failure also suffers from moderate developmental delay, congenital deafness, short stature, and a severe behavior disorder. His parents have decided not to pursue transplantation and to discontinue dialysis. He is difficult to communicate with and acts out during clinic visits, making examinations impossible.

   Under what conditions might this be an appropriate decision?

   If the medical staff disagreed with the parents, should they obtain a court order for treatment?

5. A 15-year-old girl has failed therapy for rhabdomyosarcoma, which is now widely disseminated to her lungs. Her parents, realizing that she will likely die within several weeks, want to avoid a code by developing, with their physician, specific orders for resuscitative measures. However, when the doctor inquires about discussing these decisions with their daughter, they request that this not be done, as it would "do more harm than good."

   Should the staff comply with the parents' wishes?

Part III. Suggested Reading

1. American Academy of Pediatrics. Joint Policy Statement. Principles of treatment of disabled infants. *Pediatrics*. 1984;73:559–560.
2. Cariano DA, Kanoti GA. Newborns with massive intestinal loss: Difficult choices. *N Engl J Med*. 1988;318:703–707.
3. Department of Health and Human Services. Child abuse and neglect prevention and treatment program. *Fed Reg*. 1985;50:14878–14901.
4. Kopelman LM, Irons TG, Kopelman AE. Neonatologists judge the "Baby Doe" regulations. *N Engl J Med*. 1988;318:677–683.
5. Miraie ED, Mahowald MB. Withholding nutrition from seriously ill newborn infants: a parents' perspective. *J Pediatr*. 1988;113:262-265.
6. *Hastings Center Report*. Special issue: imperiled newborns. 1987;17(6):5–32.
7. *Hastings Center Report*. Special issue: mercy, murder and morality: perspectives on euthanasia. 1989;19:1.
8. Murray T. The final, anticlimactic rule on Baby Doe. *Hastings Center Report*. 1985;15(3):5–9.
9. President's Commission for the Study of Ethical Problems in Medicine and Biomedical and Behavioral Research. *Deciding to forego life-sustaining treatment*. Chapter 6: Seriously ill newborns, 1983.
10. Rachels J. *The End of Life*. Oxford: Oxford University Press; 1986.
11. Todres ID, Guillemin J, Grodin MA, Batten D. Life-saving therapy for newborns. A questionnaire survey in the State of Massachusetts. *Pediatrics*. 1988;81:643–649.

Part IV
Doing Research:
Can Children Be Volunteered?

CHAPTER 13

Guidelines for Research

"Is this Dr. Stickman? This is Mrs. Osgood. I'm chairperson of the school committee. We have something we'd like to ask your advice about."

"Glad to help, if I can."

"We've been approached by Apex Pharmaceuticals. They have developed a new vaccine against infectious mononucleosis and would like to test it on the students here at Midtown Junior High, which would be one of 20 test sites around the country. As part of the program, the company will pay the salary of a full-time nurse for the whole school year and will donate some pieces of clinic equipment to the school. What do you think?"

How should one decide about using children for medical research?

Discussion Questions

1. What are the ethical guidelines for research with children?

2. Are preventive measure therapeutic or nontherapeutic? What are the ethical differences?

3. Who may consent for the child?

The idea of "experimenting" on children conjures up vivid pictures of Frankensteinian monsters. There is also the wholly acceptable image, however, of kindergarteners in Connecticut bravely smiling at the cameras as they proudly hold out their arms for community-wide trials of the Salk polio vaccine.

Research using children as subjects is a necessary evil, and this should be clear to any pediatrician who has had to prescribe drugs never before tested on children and in dosages arrived at only by extrapolation from adults. It would be unethical not to allow testing on children, but the history of medical research presents enough examples of truly unethical behavior, including the notorious abuses of medicine under Hitler, to make people cautious about the conditions under which research with children may be conducted.

In hospitals, consideration of the ethics of research is accomplished by Institutional Review Boards (IRBs), which generally rely on federal guidelines. Outside of that context, pediatricians may be approached by commercial drug companies that would like access to patients in a private practice or to a larger population of children, as in Midtown Junior High School. Thus, they must know what questions to ask to determine the acceptability of proposed research.

Guidelines

The following discussion is based on the guidelines set by the National Commission for the Protection of Human Subjects, which have been in effect as federal regulations since 1979.

1. Does the research address a significant question and is it well designed and likely to produce usable results? Only projects that promise valid, nontrivial results justify the time, inconvenience, and possible risk to children.

2. Has it previously been tested on animals, adults, and older children? The vulnerability of young children and infants and their inability to consent for themselves require the special protection of being last to be tested, when possible.

3. Is there benefit to the child subject? Are the risks balanced against possible benefits? Risk should be kept minimal by using the safest procedures possible, consistent with the research design, and by using information already available from treatment or diagnostic procedures when possible.

If the research poses more than minimal risk, there must be corresponding promise of benefit to the subject, and the risk may be no greater than the risk posed by available alternative treatments. In therapeutic research, when direct benefit is expected, greater risk is justified than if no benefit to that child is expected, that is, in nontherapeutic research.

If greater than minimal risk is posed by research not promising direct benefit to the subjects, it is allowable if it presents experience roughly commensurate with their experiences outside the research context, will lead to generalizable knowledge about their disorder or condition, and is of vital importance for understanding that condition. These requirements rule out nontherapeutic research on normal children which poses anything greater than minimal risk. They do allow for non-therapeutic research on normal children if the risk is only minimal.

The question of whether or not parents can "volunteer" their children for research is open to debate (see Chapter 15). Parental consent is sufficient if the research is therapeutic and the benefits obtainable only in a research context, for it would be like consenting to treatment for the child.

One view concerning nontherapeutic research argues that since children cannot consent for themselves, their participation can never be voluntary and since no direct benefit is expected, it is always unethical. Others argue that all people, including children, have a duty to contribute to society, and thus their participation in nontherapeutic medical research within appropriate limits is ethical.

When nontherapeutic research is approved, parental permission is still necessary, but assent from children over 7 years old is also required by the guidelines. These children thus have veto power over their participation. All of the other usual provisions for informed consent apply. In addition, in all kinds of research there must be opportunity to withdraw from participation at any time—at parental discretion if therapeutic, at the child's pleasure if nontherapeutic.

Preventive Measures

How do these guidelines apply to the present case? Suppose that Dr. Stickman is satisfied that the proposed study is well designed and that tests on animals and adults indicate efficacy and safety. Yet, injections are invasive procedures carrying their own risk of harm; vaccines often cause at least sore arms for a day or two, and there is always the small risk of more serious complications in at least some of the recipients. The specific effects on children are unknown, so all in all the risk factor is not negligible.

Dr. Stickman must next balance the risk against possible benefit. How likely is a child to contract a serious case of mononucleosis? If the disease is common enough, a preventive measure could be considered therapeutic research, in which case more than minimal risks could be balanced by the possible benefits. But if the risk of contracting it is very low, or the disease generally mild, then the research could not be considered of clear benefit to the children, and only a very low risk could be justified.

Consent

Suppose that Dr. Stickman judges that the research is justified in terms of risks and benefits. There is then the question of how it is to be carried out to conform to the ethical demands of informed consent. Given the marginal therapeutic value to these children of the vaccine, if it proves effective, and given their age, both parental permission and child assent should be obtained.

Who should be asked first? Participating in research should be entirely voluntary and that means freely choosing without coercion of any kind. If the children as a group are approached first by the researchers, will peer pressure be a factor? Might those who decline be taunted by accusations of being "fraidy cats" or "chicken"? If parents are approached first, they might try to put pressure on their children to participate. And if the school board is enticed by the windfall of a nurse's salary and free equipment, they in turn might try to entice the parents and children into cooperating. But then, is enticement the same as coercion?

In addition, principles of justice require that the burdens of society be fairly distributed. If advancement of knowledge in pediatrics is a desirable goal for society, then research on children is necessary. But constant vigilance is needed to ensure that it be accomplished with regard to efficiency, safety, voluntariness, and fairness. Those most vulnerable, for example, children in institutions, wards of the state, and so forth, should not ordinarily be used as research subjects. Thus, it is entirely appropriate, given proper controls, that ordinary school populations such as Midtown Junior High be enrolled. Some would say that such a program provides additional benefits by teaching valuable lessons in altruism.

CHAPTER 14

Research as Therapy

"Now that you know that it's acute leukemia, you have to decide where you want to take your son for treatment."

"What are the choices, doctor?"

"There are two possibilities. You can go to the center at the university, where they will put him on the latest research protocol. Or, you could go to one of the private oncologists, who will "tailor" therapy just for him."

"That's a hard choice. The university has the newest in the field, but we don't want our child to become a guinea pig in some big impersonal test project. The private oncologist would just be concerned with giving him the best treatment. Wouldn't that be better?"

What are the ethical issues when therapy and research come together?

Discussion Questions

1. Should "tailoring" standard treatment be considered research?

2. What are some of the problems with innovative therapy?

3. Can research be the best therapy?

Physicians who promise to design variations on standard therapy to meet the needs of a particular child may be promising too much. What they propose to do may come close to the limits of what is ethical. Although in medicine it is often true that the latest is the best, it must be demonstrated to be the best by strict standards of scientific method. Innovative therapy is not designed to meet the same strict standards.

In theory, it is possible to draw a clear distinction between practice and research. Clinical practice has the primary goal of benefiting the patient and it uses therapy that has reasonable promise of success because it is either proven, that is, validated according to the criteria of scientific study, or standard, that is, historically accepted. An historically accepted practice may be reclassified as nonvalidated when evidence appears that casts doubt on its efficacy or safety.

Research, by contrast, takes its primary goal to be testing hypotheses and contributing to generalizable knowledge. Research is considered therapeutic if it promises benefit to subjects as well as contributing to knowledge, and nontherapeutic when no benefit to subjects is expected.

Innovative Therapy and Its Problems

Distinctions blur, however, with the concept of innovative therapy or nonvalidated practice: as a form of clinical practice, its primary goal is to benefit the patient, but unlike such practice, it does not rely exclusively on scientific or historical evidence. Innovative therapy, especially in the case of leukemia, may seem perfectly acceptable since there is uncertainty with all cancer treatments. There are, however, serious problems with a too-easy acceptance of a single physician's tinkering with accepted practice.

First: reasoning, even when based on past clinical experience, may fall prey to a number of systematic fallacies. For example, studies have shown that recent experiences, especially negative ones, weigh more heavily than they should statistically. Thus, after seeing an anaphylactic reaction to a particular drug, a physician may not prescribe it again for a long time, even though it has been used successfully in the past and even if it would be the best for the patient. Hunches, guesses, and bright ideas about how to improve outcome depend on luck as much as experience, and whether luck will turn out to be bad or good cannot be predicted. In any case, relying on luck is no way to practice good medicine or ethical medicine.

Second: a physician who "tailors" standard therapy is asking the patient to take a risk. Risk taking can be justified only if there is good reason to predict that the benefits will outweigh the harms, and only experience that is scientifically grounded can be the foundation of that prediction. Innovative therapy in most cases does not meet the standards that would justify the risk.

There are other reasons to be morally skeptical. One is that the treatment may not work, and if that happens, harm is done by depriving the patient of the opportunity to benefit from validated or standard therapy. A second is that since nonvalidated practice is conducted in the context of practice, the patient is not likely to realize that it is nonvalidated; thus, the strict ethical requirements of disclosure and informed consent that apply to research may be bypassed.

Treatment may ethically be tailored to individual patients under some circumstances, however. If two treatments have been validated as equally effective, then physician and parents or child may choose one in accordance with their preferences. Also, in emergency situations one may have to improvise, but it is often ethically acceptable to act in emergencies in ways that would not be acceptable in normal circumstances.

If there is no successful validated or standard treatment, then innovation has a role, but should be limited to those regimens that have some scientific justification. In addition, parents should be fully informed and give consent, as if it were a research study. When time and conditions permit, the better course would be to turn the experiment into a full-fledged research project.

There are a number of reasons for preferring controlled research protocols over an individual physician's innovative treatment. Some of these are purely practical. For example, only research centers may be permitted to have access to the newest investigational drugs. With more patients and much wider experience with the disease and its treatment, physicians and nurses will be likely to note more quickly both problems and success. Such centers are likely to have superior support services, which can offer psychosocial support to child and family. Last but not least, they provide contact with and the support of others suffering from the same disease. This has proven to be educational as well as helpful in both practical and emotional ways.

Some of the disadvantages are practical as well. Usually research centers are at a greater distance, with increased expenses, many of which are not covered by medical insurance, and place an additional emotional burden on the family of establishing relationships with new and unfamiliar care-givers.

The moral question boils down to this: Can research therapy be the best therapy? Or, to spell it out more fully: assuming that one should always choose what is in the child's best interest, it is necessary to justify a recommendation for a child to participate in research therapy by showing that it is the best available therapy.

Research as the Best Therapy

In the case of randomized clinical trials of cancer drugs, a good case can be made in favor of research therapy. All randomized trials fulfill the requirement for scientifically valid method, promising usable results, but some kinds of trials may be more ethical than others. This can be shown by analyzing the ways the trials are conducted.

Randomized trials use two groups of subjects: those receiving the new drug or treatment and a control group, but there are three ways these trials can be carried out.

1. The trials may seek comparisons between the new treatment and no treatment. In one kind of trial the control group receives only a placebo. There are moral questions about this, especially in therapeutic research, which subjects enter in search of treatment.

2. The trial may compare those receiving the new treatment to historical outcomes, usually of subjects who remained untreated because no treatment was available. This is not morally problematic, but it is often impossible or difficult to achieve useful results.

3. The two groups may be those receiving the new treatment versus those receiving the best treatment known to date.

Most clinical trials of cancer drugs approximate the third kind, and the investigators may honestly say that they do not know which of the two treatments is best. Or, to put it another way; each child, whether randomized to the new or to the older, known treatment, has an equal chance of getting "the best." The system is fair, since the expectation of success and risk is the same for both groups and there is no rational way of deciding between them. Randomization, like a lottery, is a fair way of assigning risks and benefits. In this case, then, research therapy is the best therapy.

CHAPTER 15

"Volunteering" Well Children

"I'll take just a minute of your time, doctor. I represent the Dandy Diaper Co., and we're lining up a number of pediatricians in town who are willing to enlist parents of their infant patients to take part in a study of the toxicity and effectiveness of a new kind of diaper. It's impregnated with a new compound that we hope will decrease the incidence of severe diaper rash. The parents will be given free diapers plus a small monetary sum weekly in exchange for using our diapers regularly and keeping a record of rashes. The pediatricians will be given payment for their time and effort, of course. They will keep records and examine and treat any serious rashes that occur, and their names will be listed on any scientific publications that result."

"How safe is this new product?"

"It's been tested on young adults including some with sensitive skin and no significant side effects occurred."

Under what conditions is it all right for pediatricians to cooperate with research projects using their own patients?

Discussion Questions

1. How might pediatricians' participation in research projects with their own patients be problematic?

2. What are some reasons for thinking that well children may be volunteered for research?

3. Is it unethical for parents or physicians to be paid by the company?

Commercial companies can seduce pediatricians and parents alike with the excitement of participation in the pursuit of scientific knowledge and with promise of material rewards as well. The babies whose bodies are used in the research may or may not ever share in the same intellectual and material rewards.

Practitioners as Researchers

Are there any ethical issues about practicing pediatricians' participation in this project? Many people worry about doctors wearing two hats at the same time. Will their role as researchers interfere with their role as the babies' doctors? Might their concern for the welfare of the individual infant be temporized by the requirements of their role as researchers? May their judgment, even unwittingly, be affected by their other interests? Granted that this is always a possibility, is it likely to happen?

The authority and status of physicians may in this case work against them. Despite their explicit disclaimers to patients—"It doesn't matter a bit to me whether you decide to sign up for this or not"—parents are influenced by the mere fact of their doctor's involvement. "Well, our baby's doctor would never even suggest it if it could be harmful to her." Or a bit more naively, "They must be good, if our doctor is giving them out in his office." Conducting the research under the physician's auspices is a tacit recommendation of the project and the product.

There is also the factor of parents trying to keep on the good side of their baby's pediatrician. They might say to themselves, "If he asks me, he wants me to do it. So, I'd better do it"; or, "He'll be extra nice to us if we participate."

Parents are probably right in their calculations. Their participation may buy them a little more attention for their baby or time for their questions. In a way, it puts physicians in debt to parents: as researchers they have, so to speak, asked a favor of the parents and parents may now ask a favor in return. It changes the doctor-parent relationship in subtle ways.

It is not always a bad thing to change a doctor-patient relationship. Enlisting parents in a research project promotes a sense of partnership and cooperation between parents and physician. It empowers the parents and enhances their sense of their own worth. So, pediatricians who are uncomfortable with the traditional imbalance of power and authority between physicians and patients may welcome a chance to improve it. Participating in a research project also helps educate parents about the nature of medical knowledge, both the carefulness with which research is conducted and the inherent element of uncertainty in medical practice. It makes them more intelligent users of medical services and better advocates for their children.

The more serious argument against having pediatricians who are also researchers is that their dual role may compromise the care of the child. Physician-researchers might urge a certain product or procedure on the parents that they would not otherwise recommend, and in the event of tentative negative findings, they may be more reluctant to switch the babies off the experimental diaper until the project has achieved its objective, that is, until significant differences have been demonstrated.

All of these negative effects may happen even if the physicians' only interest in the research is scientific. They will have dual loyalty if they have involvement with commercial research projects.

"Volunteering" Well Children

There is a further problem. Insofar as the research into new and better diapers is conducted for the primary purpose of gaining new knowledge, and its goal is not to improve the health of the already healthy babies, it is classified as nontherapeutic research. The general principle that applies to research with children is that the risk/benefit ratio must be favorable (see Chapter 13). If no benefit is expected for the babies, then even if there is virtually no risk some other way of justifying it must be found and the project should be approached with great caution.

The AAP has stated that benefits to society may not constitute justification for drug testing of healthy children, even if there is a great need for information. The Academy goes on to suggest that this need may be met by conducting tests on ill children who can be expected to benefit from it. Sometimes, though, the information required can be obtained only from healthy children. Is there no ethical way this research can be carried out?

Some people would answer no. There are two reasons for this: 1) the research promises no benefit to the babies, and research on children when the risk is not outweighed by possible benefit is not ethical, and 2) young children cannot consent for themselves and any nontherapeutic research without voluntary consent is unethical.

Now, consider the other side. Are there any good reasons to be offered that could justify parents' volunteering their healthy children for research? Can the negative arguments be answered? Two kinds of responses are possible. The first is to argue that all citizens, children included, have an obligation to contribute to the social welfare. When certain kinds of research can be conducted only on young children or infants, then, with proper control of risk and with appropriate informed consent from parents, children may be "volunteered."

The second kind of response to the arguments against allowing healthy children as subjects in nontherapeutic research attempt to show some benefit that may accrue to the subjects. All babies, after all, are the potential victims of diaper rash. So, those who contribute to the development of diapers that prevent the rash will be potential beneficiaries as well. The strength of this argument depends on the incidence of the condition being researched. If the disease is highly contagious and serious, for example, polio, then the potential benefit to the subjects if greater than if the likelihood and seriousness of contracting it is very slight. In the case of severe diaper rash, the incidence is low, the example a bit far-fetched, and so this argument would not carry much weight.

There may be indirect benefits, however. When the children are older, they will learn that they participated as babies in a scientific research study and can take pride in it. Thus, they will be learning good attitudes toward altruism and civic duty and will have cause for enhanced self-esteem.

A further argument can be made, however, by comparing the possible right of parents to volunteer their children for research to parents' rights in other areas. Parents are allowed to "use" children in various ways for the benefit of the whole family, and what is a benefit to the whole family is also a benefit to the child involved. For example, parents may sign child movie stars or infant TV stars to commercial contracts and allow them to be employed, without the child's informed consent. Within appropriate limits, these activities are considered acceptable and not exploitative and the risk or inconvenience of using a new diaper product is not likely to be greater than the discomfort of acting under bright lights or the psychological stress of being in the public eye. If the comparison holds, then parents may volunteer their children and physicians need not feel that they are proposing anything unethical by presenting the option for appropriately screened research projects to parents.

Payment

There remains the question of payment to the family and to the physician. If a family is in extreme poverty, then even a modest payment can be coercive. For this reason some people say that populations that are especially susceptible to coercion or exploitation, including those in extreme poverty, especially in the Third World, prisoners, the homeless, and institutionalized children should never be used as research subjects. For both family and physician, payment may also seem coercive or corruptive if it is out of proportion to the time, inconvenience, and risk involved. A good test for physicians might be whether or not they would be embarrassed to reveal to the families the extent of their own rewards. In general, payments that are likely to influence people to do things they would rather not do, that is, rewards that are "too good to pass up," would be unethical.

CHAPTER 16

Psychological Research

"Could I just ask you a quick question on the phone, doctor? I just got a note from Lizzie's day care center asking our permission for her to be a research subject. A team of psychologists wants to come in and interview all the 3-year-olds and observe them at play and make videotapes. They're interested in finding out about aggressive behavior in normal kids. It sounds OK, but do you think I should sign it? Can it do Lizzie any harm?"

Are there special ethical concerns about psychological research?

Discussion Questions

1. Are there ethically relevant differences between psychological research and other research?

2. Is psychological research important enough to justify the risks? Are there some things we will never be able to find out because of ethical constraints on research?

3. What are some ethically responsible steps researchers could take to increase informed, voluntary consent and assent?

Even the most trusting or sophisticated parents might be put off by researchers' request to include their 3-year-old in such a study. Parents probably do not want to think of sweet, innocent young children as exhibiting aggressive behavior, and even if they are willing to entertain the idea in general because they have read some psychology in college, they may not want to think about it in relation to their own child. To ask the question may already be to raise their anxiety or to change ever so slightly their perception of their child. Psychological research often poses questions of a sensitive nature, which may make it immediately more difficult to enroll subjects than in other kinds of research.

For parents who are not so easily put off by the idea of investigating areas of sensitivity, but are nevertheless appropriately concerned with their child's welfare, the first challenge to the researcher is likely to be, "Well, how will it affect Lizzie? Could it be harmful to her to bring up questions about hitting, punching, or biting? Will it focus her attention on it or make her ashamed of behavior that her family accepts as pretty ordinary?"

The honest researcher may need to answer many of these concerns by saying, "I don't think it will be harmful or change her behavior at all, but we really don't know." And herein lies one of the most serious ethical difficulties in the conduct of psychological research. Because of the complex nature of human behavior and because psychology is a newer science, we cannot predict with reliability how individuals will respond in specific situations. Granted, every medical research project deals with the unknown, but in the areas of thought, attitudes, and behavior, predicting risk with any degree of probability is much more difficult.

The dilemma thus is this: in order for parents to have the information they need in order to give informed consent, the researcher needs to be able to make a dependable risk assessment. Lack of previous research results in a lack of information about risks. But to ask parents to give consent without relevant information—or even, it could be argued, to propose to carry out research when one does not oneself know the risk of harm to the subjects—is unethical. Thus, there is a self-perpetuating set of difficulties seemingly more irresolvable in psychological research than in other kinds of medical research.

Perhaps this point about ignorance of risk exaggerates the problem. Suppose that Lizzie's parents are convinced of her steadiness of mind and willing to sign her up to be observed and interviewed. They understand that the purpose of the study is to establish a norm of certain kinds of behavior. Suppose, then, that the investigator finds that Lizzie places at the high scale of aggressive behavior and perhaps in her interview exhibits a higher than average level of anxiety about it. What is the researcher's obligation to the child and parents? Should all the parents receive anonymous results of all the research? Should Lizzie's parents be told her particular scores? Should the researcher contact them with her concerns about Lizzie? Should the research study have provisions for intervention, and if so, should it be immediate or follow-up? Other medical research has provision for treatment or compensation in case of injury; how should such injury be handled in psychological studies? Given the way society often misuses psychological labeling and reports of treatment, one might argue that the possible harms of psychological research could be greater and more long-lasting as well as less likely to be foreseen than other kinds of research.

There are other ways in which the ethical requirements of research appear to throw up obstacles to psychological research in particular. Much of what is important to know involves establishing setting of norms, and this requires the participation of large numbers of well children. Such research by its very nature is nontherapeutic and, by the provision of the federal regulations governing research with children, requires not only parental permission but the child's own assent as well for children older than 7 years. For those old enough to be consulted, the child who says no has absolute veto power over his or her participation, even if parents consent (see Chapter 13). Given the sometimes whimsical nature of children's cooperation, their interests and loyalties, it often may happen that baseball will win out over boring interviews. Even in therapeutic research the child's cooperation is required in psychological or psychiatric studies in a different way and to a greater degree than a treatment for physical ailments.

For teenagers, confidentiality in research poses special problems. Can researchers guarantee to keep information from parents, and can they hope to get accurate information about sexuality, drug use, and other sensitive issues if they do not?

Importance

Against these legitimate concerns about ethical restraints on research, the case for the importance of psychological research, broadly defined, can be made. There are at least four major areas where much needs to be learned.

1. Drug therapy for conditions such as depression, which seem to be increasing in incidence and appearing in younger and younger children.

2. Clarifying diagnostic categories and criteria and determining the efficacy of drug versus behavioral versus environmental control of the so-called syndrome of hyperactivity or minimal brain dysfunction.

3. Learning more about the attitudes and behavior associated with many social problems such as substance abuse, sexually transmitted disease, teen pregnancy, and suicide in children and teens with the goal of developing effective means of prevention.

4. Establishing and updating norms of psychological and social functioning. For example, are children's lives really affected by fears of nuclear war? What is the effect of infant day care on the later development of the child? How are children of divorce or one-parent families or homosexual families or working mothers different from those brought up in the "Leave It to Beaver" tradition?

Steps Toward Ethical Research

There well may be important questions that should remain unanswered because there are no ethically acceptable ways to do the research. We cannot and will not subject children to controlled studies that change radically whatever is current in family structure and child-rearing methods.

However, researchers can try to be thoughtful and creative in designing research projects to protect children and yet make it attractive to both the children and their parents. To counter fears about confidentiality, for example, one could collect data with pertinent demographic information, but without making it possible to identify individuals. This makes it impossible to offer therapeutic intervention if such a need is discovered, which is a common objection to anonymous AIDS testing of adults, but that may be a reasonable trade-off to encourage teens to supply much needed information. Where it is legal to allow treatment of teens without parental permission, researchers could try to have it made legal to conduct research in the same way.

For younger children, perhaps the opposite is needed. Lizzie's parents could be offered the results of a general screening test, something that could be of benefit to them, just as the subjects in the long-term Framingham heart study were offered free physical exams and monitoring over the years, probably better than many of them would have secured for themselves. For the child who might choose baseball over the time spent in an interview, the researcher may have to sell children on the idea that this is a way to find out what scientists do, or if appropriate, a way to find out more about themselves. To be an interview subject could be seen as a badge of honor to boast to one's friends about, rather than a waste of good play time. None of this is unethical as long as it is an honest appraisal of what the researcher is doing and is presented without coercion.

Part IV. Additional Cases for Discussion

1. The parents of a newborn with anencephaly wish to have the child's organs used for research, so that "the child's life will have some value."

    What criteria, if any, would provide good moral reasons for allowing such procedures?

2. A 10-year-old child has suffered several relapses of leukemia, and all modes of standard therapy have been exhausted. The hospital specialist offers to enroll the child on a Phase I/II study. It uses a new drug currently being tested in adults but with virtually no track record in pediatrics. The parents say they will try anything to avoid "giving-up." "Even if it doesn't work with your child, what we learn might help some child someday," notes the researcher.

    As a member of the Institutional Review Board, what should be the requirements to approve such research?

    Should it be considered therapeutic or nontherapeutic research?

3. A researcher wishes to test a vaccine against rotovirus. She proposes to administer the vaccine to half of her normal infant subjects and give a placebo injection to the other half.

    What ethical issues are involved in the use of an experimental and control group?

    What measures can be taken to ensure that the benefits and harms are fairly distributed among the subjects?

Part IV. Suggested Reading

1. Department of Health and Human Services. Rules and Regulations 45 CFR 46: Revised as of March 8, 1983. Subpart A: Basic HHS Policy for Protection of Human Research Subjects; Subpart D: Additional Protections for Children Involved as Subjects in Research. Reprinted in: Levine RJ. Children. In:*Ethics and Regulation of Clinical Research,* 2nd ed., Baltimore-Munich: Urban & Schwarzenberg; 1986.
2. Grodin MA, Alpert JJ. Children as participants in medical research. *Pediatr Clin N Am.* 1988;35(6):1389–1401.
3. Holder AR. Chapter VI: The minor as research subject or transplant donor. In: *Legal Issues in Pediatrics and Adolescent Medicine*, 2nd ed., New Haven: Yale University Press; 1985.
4. Kapp MB. Children's assent for participation in pediatric research protocols. *Clin Pediatr.* 1983;22(4):275–278.
5. Levine RJ. Chapter 10: Children. In: *Ethics and Regulation of Clinical Research*, 2nd ed., Baltimore-Munich: Urban & Schwarzenberg; 1986.
6. McCormick R. Proxy consent in the experimental situation. *Perspectiv Biol Med.* 1974;18(1):2–20. Reprinted in: Beauchamp TL, Walters L (eds): *Contemporary Issues in Bioethics*, 2nd ed. Belmont, Calif: Wadsworth Publishing Company; 1982:549–557.
7. Ramsey P. The patient as person. New Haven: Yale University Press; 1970:11–17. Reprinted in: Beauchamp TL, Walters L (eds): *Contemporary Issues in Bioethics*, 2nd ed. Belmont, Calif: Wadsworth Publishing Company; 1982:546–549.
8. Weithorn LA. Children's capacities to decide about participation in research. *IRB, Rev Hum Subj.* 1983;5(2):1–5.

Part V
Relating to Patients:
What Is the Best Doctor-Patient
Relationship?

CHAPTER 17

The Virtuous Physician

"Excuse me. May I sit here? I'm Milton Mendes. I'm new on staff."

"Ed Cutter here. Been at Memorial longer than anyone can remember. Seen lots of good people come and go. Some not so good ones, too."

"I wonder what it is that makes a doctor good. You know, I didn't go into medicine just to be technically excellent and financially successful. I want to be a good doc, in the fullest sense."

"Well, there are lots of lofty moral principles, professional codes, and medical-legal guidelines. They will tell you what's right and keep you out of trouble, but if you want my opinion, to become a good physician, find yourself a good model and follow that person's lead."

Is this good advice?

Discussion Questions

1. To be a good physician, is it enough to do what is right? Must one also be a good person? What is the difference?

2. How does one become a good person?

3. Should physicians be held to higher moral standards than other people?

The usual approach to ethics asks, What should I do? A different approach asks, What kind of person should I be? The latter kind of theory focuses on character traits or virtues and has its roots in Aristotle, who often uses the practice of medicine as a paradigm of professions and roles in society.

Aristotle develops the concept of practically wise persons, those who embody the virtues that society admires. Their character is such that they act virtuously, as it were by habit: they have trained themselves always to act with courage, temperance, justice, and so on. They are the ideal of morally good persons.

Doing right versus being good

Aristotle's theory offers no list of moral rules to follow, for none is needed. For the virtuous persons, their own good judgment and a steady disposition to do the good lead them to knowing and doing what is right in any situation. Morality is not a matter of rules; doing what is right depends on sizing up the situation, appraising the possibilities, finding the golden mean—for moderation and balance were the mark of all virtues for Aristotle—and then doing it.

Aristotle goes on to define happiness as the disposition of the soul to choose in accordance with virtue, meaning that the good life is the happy life, that virtue is its own reward in the sense of internal well-being. Because morality is a matter of good character and the happiness it is expected to bring provides an incentive for being virtuous, there is no gap between knowing the good and doing it.

For Aristotle, virtue and good character depend on practical reason, and only rational persons can be virtuous. Like Aristotle, more modern definitions connect virtue to well-being by saying that virtues are the human qualities necessary and desirable for human flourishing in communities.

A quick look at the specific virtues that Aristotle recommends suggests that some changes are in order to fit contemporary life. Remember, virtues are character traits that a society admires. For Aristotle's male-oriented Athenian society, courage, temperance, justice, and magnanimity were appropriate. Interpreting these rather broadly, for instance, supposing that justice includes honesty, makes these perfectly appropriate still. However, for today's ideal, especially for the ideal of the virtuous doctor, one would want to add compassion, sympathy, and benevolence. In terms of moral theory, this is adding what Hume calls "the passions" to the Greek rationalist ideal. It also helps satisfy some of the feminist critique of the Western tradition in moral philosophy by placing value on feelings as well as intellect.

The best known contemporary proponent of virtue theory suggests that it is because modern society has no consensus on values that moral rules and principles have been developed to guide decisions and actions. This has not proven successful, however, for a pluralistic society will offer differing rules and thus cannot resolve conflicts.

The alternative is to focus on the virtues instead of rules, and to work consciously to build consensus on values and a sense of community. Applied to medicine, this might mean consensus both within the medical community and within the broader community, that is, shared expectations for the virtues of the good physician and the nature of the doctor–patient relationship.

According to this view, the virtues of one's professional role should not be isolated from the other roles a person plays in society. Physicians may also be parents, citizens, neighbors, friends; but whatever virtues are called for by those roles should be consistent with one another. Individuals must view themselves as whole persons. One could not be both a good pediatrician and a child molester. The so-called Nazi doctors who used medicine for genocide and torture cannot be called good doctors. Thus, according to this view, one cannot be a good doctor and a bad person.

Becoming a Good Person

How does a person become a good person? Can virtues be taught? Aristotle's answer is a good one, that one becomes virtuous by modeling oneself on a person recognized as virtuous: noticing what that person does, practicing acting that way, internalizing the disposition to act that way, and finally, establishing that way of acting as a habit or character trait. Becoming a virtuous person requires a kind of apprenticeship and role modeling.

There are indeed similarities between learning to be a virtuous person and learning to be a good doctor. Much of medical education is based on the same assumptions: one learns by doing and by following the model of a good practitioner.

Moral Standards

There remains the question of how virtuous the physician must be. If one is following rules, then there is a distinction between what is required and what goes beyond the required. To do more than is required is referred to as supererogatory. Thus, the shady character who says, "I have done just what the rule says; I need not do anything more" is technically correct.

Is it enough to avoid doing wrong? It would be nice to think that ethics could be reduced to one golden rule or even 10 bronze commandments, but moral theories that rest on rules or principles have the effect of encouraging a minimalist attitude: "Ah, this is the rule. All I have to do is just what it says to do or avoid what it says is wrong, and I have fulfilled my duty completely. No one can fault me for not doing more." Rule-based thinking can also encourage a legalistic approach: to act within the letter of the law, but not necessarily in its spirit.

It is difficult to defend the view that physicians should be held to higher standards than other people. The argument usually given is that privilege and power brings responsibility; those who have had the privilege of medical education and enjoy the status of physician have greater responsibility than others. This might work as a reason for the physician being a good Samaritan or doing the equivalent of legal pro bono work, but it does not speak to the issue of being a good person. Another good reason for holding physicians to a very high moral standard is because of the potential their work carries for doing harm. The public need not worry so much about the moral character of those who play minor roles in society or whose work has little effect on others; as accountability and concern go up, however, the greater the impact that a person's life and work can have on others. Moreover, since physicians have a great deal of autonomy in their work, others need to be able to depend on their integrity and good character.

There are also very practical reasons for insisting on high moral character for physicians. If a person is willing to cheat in the non-professional part of one's life, it becomes easier to be willing to cheat in professional work as well. Relying on moral rules may allow compartmentalization of life; insisting on good moral character overall does not allow this, for the person of good character acts virtuously by habit. Acting virtuously is part of the very nature and being of the person of good character.

The importance of good character is recognized by the American Board of Pediatrics. The Verification of Clinical Competence Form requires the training program director to certify candidates for board examination to have "moral and ethical integrity." It furthers specifies respect for patient's right of privacy, demonstration of a caring attitude toward patients and families, and demonstration of personal honesty.

CHAPTER 18

Loyalty to Parents

"Stand up and let's take a look at you. What are these bruises back here, Natalie?"

"It's not her fault, Dr. Needleman. I'm responsible. I've been under such a lot of stress this month. My wife has just left me and the children. It was a shock. And I lost my temper for one minute the other day. I am so sorry."

"This sounds serious."

"It will never happen again. I wanted to ask if you know about any groups for single parents I could join, just to talk things over. You won't have to tell anyone about this, will you? Natalie knows I love her and wouldn't ever hurt her."

"I am certainly willing to do what I can to help. I've known your family a long time. But, this does look like a problem."

What are the doctor's responsibilities to parents, to child, and to the state?

Discussion Questions

1. What is the foundation of and limits of the pediatrician's loyalty to parents?

2. How should pediatricians balance their obligations to parents, child, and the state?

3. Is it ever justified for pediatricians to break the law in order to protect parents from charges of child abuse or neglect?

The doctor–patient relationship is built on mutual trust. Parents' trust in the pediatrician promotes honesty, cooperation, and the confidence to accept the medical help their child needs. Physicians' trust in parents promotes a partnership between them, with the goal of helping the child. The role of parents in actually providing medical care has become especially important in recent years, with the move toward shorter hospital stays and more extensive home care.

Usually the relationship of mutual trust works well, but it is put to the test when the pediatrician suspects child abuse or neglect or in other ways encounters conflicts between loyalty to parents, responsibility for the well-being of the child, and obligations to the state. To help resolve these conflicts it is helpful to review the reasons why pediatricians owe loyalty to parents and to raise questions about possible limits on that loyalty. When are pediatricians' obligations to parents legitimately overridden by other obligations?

The pediatrician's first loyalty is to the child. Pediatricians owe loyalty to parents by virtue of their status as guardians of their children. On an older view, people would have said that God has given parents guardianship over their children. On a more modern view, parents' status is conferred by the state, which has taken upon itself ultimate responsibility for the well-being of all of its citizens. When parents do not fulfill their responsibility, they lose their status as guardians and thus lose their claim to the loyalty of physicians.

Situations that present clear and imminent serious danger to the child's life or well-being, whether posed by parents directly or by conditions that the parents cannot correct, demand that pediatricians put into motion whatever is required to protect their child. If the danger can be avoided only by separating child from parents, then it must be done.

If physicians' first loyalty in cases of clear danger is to the child, their second loyalty in such cases is to the state. This is because the whole of the state's claim to loyalty is founded on the responsibility it takes for children. If the parents fail to protect and nurture the child, and the pediatrician is in the front line in discovering this, then he or she has a straightforward obligation to report this to the state.

Only third loyalty is to the parents, which is to say that loyalty to parents or parents' welfare should never override responsibility to the child when danger is clear and imminent. In the normal cases or in cases where the danger is not clear, loyalty is owed to parents because of the crucial role they play in their child's development.

Reporting Parents

Among the clear cases of danger to a child, those involving cultural and religious differences deserve special mention. Beliefs of Jehovah's Witnesses and Christian Scientists pose a possible counter-example to the principle that pediatricians should always act to protect the child. It is argued on grounds of freedom of religion and the rights of parents to choose their children's life style, including religion, that the state has no jurisdiction to require medical treatment that their religions forbid. Some states have enacted statutes to protect parents from prosecution if because of certain designated religious beliefs they fail to provide generally accepted life-saving medical care.

Despite this, courts have generally been willing to issue orders for life-saving blood transfusions for the children of Jehovah's Witnesses under the principle that one can "make a martyr of oneself, but cannot make a martyr of one's child," and Christian Scientist parents have been prosecuted for denying their children life-saving medical care.

Some cases of possible abuse or neglect are more problematic because it is not clear that serious danger is posed to the child. However, most states assume a conservative stance and require that physicians report all cases of even suspected abuse or neglect.

The phrase "suspected abuse or neglect" is ambiguous. It covers two kinds of cases. In the first, a physician discovers bruises or broken bones that cannot be accounted for. Abuse is suspected as the cause, although the parents may offer other explanations. The second kind of case is future oriented. It can be predicted that parents who refuse treatment or have not kept follow-up appointments will continue to fail to provide needed medical care for their children and therefore are suspected of neglect before it happens. Although in most areas of law people are presumed innocent until proven guilty, protection of children may require reporting and investigation before the fact.

There are a number of reasons why physicians may be reluctant to report suspected abuse or neglect. They may not be willing to give up the time and go through the hassle of court appearances. They may not want to jeopardize their relationship with the parents, especially if the evidence is slim. They may judge that the child will be better served by staying in the present situation than disrupting his or her life, especially if the foster care system is not very good. Or, physicians may trust their own judgments of particular families and feel confident that the incident will not be repeated.

However reluctant the physician, reporting laws do not allow for much discretion. If Dr. Needleman does not report Natalie's father, she will be breaking the law, for the father's admission of guilt places this case squarely in the category of abuse. However, if Dr. Needleman feels confident that the child is not in danger and sees no point in calling in the authorities, may she morally decide not to report? The only good arguments that can be given for breaking the law come under the heading of civil disobedience. Civil disobedience is defined as breaking a law that is considered to be wrong, where it is thought to be immoral to obey it. Trespassing on private property in order to free laboratory animals to protest their use in experimentation is an example of breaking the law by civil disobedience. The act of disobedience must be done publicly, nonviolently, with the purpose of having the law changed, by those willing to accept punishment for it, and only as a last resort. Lawful ways of persuading people of the immorality of the law and trying to get it changed must be exhausted first. The civil rights movement is an example of a successful use of civil disobedience.

In order for the doctor's failure to report the parent to be justified in terms of civil disobedience, she would have to begin by announcing publicly what she is doing. If her original intention was to protect the child and not jeopardize her relationship with the father, going public will certainly defeat her purpose. It is dangerous and not morally defensible to make exceptions for oneself. What if her judgment is wrong? The point of the reporting law is to open up an investigation and protect against mistaken judgments. If the state had wanted pediatricians to have sole discretion about when to report, the reporting law would be phrased to allow it.

One of the strongest arguments against civil disobedience, and one that applies here, rests on the idea of an implicit contract between the state and its citizens. In return for the benefits that a state affords people, they owe loyalty to its laws. Physicians enjoy the privileges of practicing medicine by contract, as it were, with the state. They are in turn designated by the state as protectors of children. Thus, the duty to report child abuse and neglect is a special duty of physicians and should be fulfilled as the law prescribes. Pediatricians can and should, of course, work to change laws they think are inadequate or wrong, but should do so in lawful ways.

CHAPTER 19

Saying "No"

"Am I tired! I thought 5:30 would never come. What a day this has been!"

"Then you won't want to hear about the phone call I just took for you, Dr. Smart. Oscar's family wants to meet you at the hospital this evening to talk about getting him transferred to the intensive care unit. They want more aggressive respiratory care and are being pretty insistent."

"Oh, no. Couldn't they make it in the morning? Anyway, poor Oscar isn't going to come out of his vegetative state. It's been 9 months now and if anything, they should begin thinking about tapering off treatment altogether."

When may a physician say no?

Discussion Questions

1. What limits may a physician set against demanding parents?

2. When is it permissible to refuse to comply with parents' request for treatment of their child?

3. When is it ethical to say, "No, I can't do this; it goes against my conscience"?

Medical residents get used to being awakened in the middle of the night, being on call 36 hours at a time, and having precious little time to call their own. Among various reasons offered to justify this state of affairs is that it is good preparation for the "real world" of practicing medicine. Kids do get ear aches at 3 AM, parents do wait until after working hours to panic, and a hospitalized child can take a turn for the worse just as his physician is about to head out for a game of tennis. A doctor's life is not entirely one's own. But, one might well ask, To what extent should it be?

Setting Limits

Patients do have legitimate claims on physicians' time, energy, and attention. Only a few specialities allow for a 9 to 5 schedule, and pediatrics is certainly not one of them. While most parents are considerate and reasonable, there are always some who make demands that physicians feel they have no obligation to fulfill. How to say no in a nonhurtful way is a psychological question; when to say no is an ethical one.

Discussions of the doctor–patient relationship are often framed in terms of analogies. Physicians have been compared to everything from priests to plumbers. One widely accepted model pictures the doctor and patient as parties to a contract, with duties and compensations clearly spelled out. This model has been criticized, however, for encouraging a minimalist approach: it appears to set down just what services are required, with the implication that these can be precisely determined and, when fulfilled, nothing else is required. The doctor–patient relationship is not that neat, at least not in pediatrics, and most if not all who enter the profession expect to give more of themselves than some legalistically defined minimum.

The doctor–patient relationship has also been described as a covenant, which captures the special trusting, reciprocal, and open-ended nature of the relationship and avoids the unfortunate pecuniary connotations of the contract analogy. However, a covenant relationship, like the loose bonds between friends, may make setting limits difficult.

How then can one set limits on the doctor–patient relationship? One way to think about this is that it is a matter of style. One physician wants to be as available and accommodating as humanly possible; she is always ready and willing to "go the extra mile." Another wants to be able to separate professional life from private life, arranging a work schedule that clears the decks completely for regular off-duty hours. Choices between solo or group practice, subspecialty versus general pediatrics, rural or urban areas, and so on allow individuals to decide what kind of physician they want to be (see Chapter 17).

There are other, more controversial ways of setting limits. Is it morally acceptable for a physician to decide not to treat patients with AIDS? Or not accept Medicaid patients? If the reason is purely self-interest, whether for convenience, monetary concerns, or fear, is that a good enough reason?

Conscience

The ultimate case of setting limits is to refuse parent's request to treat a child. There are two classes of cases in which physicians may want to refuse to treat:

1. Cases in which refusal is justified by the strongest possible reasons, namely that it would be bad medicine and against accepted medical practice. The reasons given in these cases are objective, not dependent on who one is as a particular person, but what any reasonable physician would subscribe to.

2. Cases in which the reasons for refusing are matters of personal conscience and thus subjective, that is, dependent on the physician's personal beliefs, values, religion, and so on. Conforming to the principle that professionals should not impose their own values on patients and families, the physician's refusal to

perform a procedure for personal reasons should not make it impossible for the patient to receive that service.

One would like to say that no one should ever have to act against conscience. But in certain circumstances this may be a luxury that society cannot afford to extend to those with special skills and training. To refuse when no alternative is available to the patient constitutes abandonment, which is both morally and legally wrong. One explanation of why the physician may not refuse rests on the theory that obligations arise out of need. To say that persons need something is to say that they will be harmed if they do not get it. Needs give rise to obligations when there is a special relationship between the person who has needs and the person who is able to fulfill those needs. A patient in need does not necessarily have a claim against every physician, but there is an obligation when a physician is the only one who can fulfill those needs, for example, being the only one available in a geographic district or the only one with, say, surgical skills.

A special case of being the only one who can fulfill a patient's needs arises from the unique nature of the doctor–patient relationship. The therapeutic relationship, the healing touch, or, more mystically, the laying on of hands, has beneficial effects, both physiological and psychological—perhaps physiological because of being psychological—that result from the attention of a known and beloved physician. This can be one of the great satisfactions of clinical practice, but the demands on one's time can become excessive when too many little ones or their parents claim, "Only Dr. Smart can make me feel better," or "I only want Dr. Smart to give me the injection." No one wants to repeat the hospital residency pattern indefinitely, with sleepless nights and no time to call one's own. But when a long-time patient needs to be seen at night, can one say no?

Saying No

The ultimate test of the physician's right to say no may come at the end of life. When parents plead, "Please do everything for my child," may the physician say no?

This appears to be a new question. Physicians in recent years have generally been committed to a "do everything policy." The cases that hit the newspapers and the courts are like the Karen Ann Quinlan case or the Baby Andrew case: parents want to stop treatment, physicians and hospitals want to continue. This commitment has been reinforced, no doubt, by the social climate that produced the Baby Doe regulations (see Chapter 9).

In the old days, it is said, physicians took it upon themselves to stop or not initiate treatment. If an infant were born severely deformed or so weak that survival was unlikely, the country doctor might not make the effort to save it or might even take more active measures to assure its death. The parents may have been told it was stillborn. In today's world of hospital records and in the moral climate of parental autonomy, such behavior seems impossible to manage and scandalous even to contemplate. There must be a middle ground between always doing everything and taking it upon oneself not to treat, and there must be principles by which to decide.

Are there, then, circumstances where the physician should take the initiative and refuse to treat? The clearest answer to this is that if the proposed treatment is both futile and inhumane, that is, causes significant suffering to the child, then it is wrong to do it. To say it is wrong is to say that there is a positive obligation to refuse. What if the treatment is futile, but causes the child no suffering or harm? Then a somewhat weaker answer can be given: there is no obligation to treat; it is permissible either to treat or not to treat, depending on circumstances. To say it is permissible means there is no obligation to do it, but it would not be wrong to do. Strictly speaking, parents cannot demand useless or inappropriate treatment. However, there might be good reasons for not refusing.

Physicians must decide concerning treatments that are neither morally required nor morally wrong what reasons will be good enough to justify treatment. The determination can be made by cost/benefit analysis. For example, one might decide to continue treating an accident victim for the parents' sake, to give them time to adjust to the idea that their child will not survive. In addition, they will then be able to carry on their parenting role, which will be of benefit to the child. Or one might decide to continue a treatment that is not effective in order to make arrangements for organ donation. In another case, one might decide not to continue futile treatment because of the high emotional cost to the nursing and resident staff and the cost in material resources.

What, then, about Oscar? Continued treatment is futile in terms of any recovery, but is presumably not harmful to the child who is in a persistent vegetative state. Thus, it could be considered not wrong. However, in the light of high emotional and material cost, it would be reasonable for the physician to take the initiative and counsel the parents against continued therapy.

CHAPTER 20

Considering Costs

"Mrs. Parente, the results of the lab tests on Pedro are back and they rule out a number of things as the cause of his headaches. But I'm still not sure what's going on with him. I'd like to refer you to a pediatric neurologist."

"That sounds like a good idea, Dr. Wise. We want the best for him. Who do you suggest? And will his bill be covered by our HMO, like yours is?"

"Let's see. I don't see the person I had in mind on the HMO list. In fact, there is no pediatric neurologist, just an adult neurologist."

"That's not as good, is it?"

"Well, an adult neurologist would be all right, but I think a pediatric specialist would be better. However, the HMO doesn't like me to refer outside their lists of member doctors. And it may cause some problems for me if I do."

How should physicians respond to various concerns about cost?

Discussion Question

1. When is it ethically appropriate for the pediatrician to consider costs?

2. What are the implications for the doctor–patient relationship of health maintenance organizations (HMOs), prepayment plans, and for-profit health-care institutions?

3   If the practice of medicine becomes a business, how will it change things?

The ideal of the practicing physician is to be able to do what is best for the patient without regard to cost. Whether this ideal ever existed in some golden days of the past or is a feasible goal to try to achieve in the future, one thing is sure: it is not the way medicine is practiced in this country today. All physicians must be concerned about cost. A crucial question is, cost to whom?

Considering Costs

HMOs are attempts to lower costs of health care to patients. They accomplish this in three ways: by spreading the risks among a large group, as in any insurance plan, by contracting for services at more favorable rates than individuals could, and by limiting services. The conditions of the contract are supposed to be known to the subscriber, who is assured good and reliable health care, but without the luxuries of choosing among a wide range of physicians and other health-care providers and facilities.

Actually, parents are often in the position of choosing among alternatives for their children based on cost: public school versus private, day care versus summer camp. Pediatricians regularly offer certain kinds of cost-conscious choices: brand-name versus generic drugs, private versus semiprivate hospital rooms. The key to considering costs for parents is to be sure that they are well informed.

If the HMO simply will not pay for specialists not on their list, it is the parents' decision to go with what the HMO allows or to cover the cost of the pediatric specialist themselves. What is important is not to be paternalistic and make the choice for them. They may have resources unknown to the physician and providing information will make them more educated consumers when it comes time to renew or change their medical insurance.

Implications for the Doctor–Patient Relationship

Although physicians are accustomed to thinking about costs to patients, HMOs introduce the necessity of thinking about costs to physicians. Working under a system of either positive or negative incentives for keeping health care costs down, physicians may be placed in the untenable position where what is good for their patients' health and pocketbooks is not good for the health of the physicians' pocketbook.

Under some systems the burden of proof is on the physician to make the case to the HMO that the specialist or extra tests are really needed. If the appeal for a pediatric neurologist is successful, the HMO will pay for it, but that will push up Dr. Wise's use of resources compared to other pediatricians in the HMO pool and she will not only have to expend considerable time and effort on extra paperwork, but may also lose a portion of the incentive pay from the HMO that she would otherwise receive. If this particular HMO has high incentives, either in terms of penalties for overutilization or bonuses for underutilization, and/or if Dr. Wise has a high percentage of HMO families in her patient population, she may lose a considerable portion of her income.

The ethical issue here is a simple conflict of interest: if the doctor works in her patients' interests, she stands to lose; if she works in her own interest, the patients stand to lose. By contrast, the simple fee-for-service system, despite other problems, has the advantage of making the physician's and the patients' interests coincide: only if the physician works for the best interest of the patient will she gain a good reputation and build up her practice. The more well cared for and satisfied her patients, the more rewards to the physician. The cost-containment policies of HMOs and for-profit organizations reverse the situation.

Even the hint of a possible conflict of interest will have impact on the doctor–patient relationship. Medicine has traditionally operated under a patient-centered ethic: the patients trust that the physician is always working for their best interest. Just as that trust is strained when the physician wears two hats as both therapist and researcher, it is strained when he or she has divided loyalty both to the best interest of the patient and to the best interest of the HMO. Is the physician employed by the patient or by the HMO? An injured workman is justified in being suspicious of the company doctor who pronounces him well enough to go back to work, and he prefers to get the go-ahead from his own doctor. Can he trust that the HMO doctor is using her own best medical judgment? Might the physician be offering treatment according to restrictions and requirements set down by third parties? Even worse, the system might encourage physicians to withhold information about treatment options.

HMOs, diagnosis-related groups (DRGs), for-profit hospitals, and other cost-containment incentives do work. Changes in physician behavior have been documented by such measures as length of hospital stay and use of lab tests. Whether or not these changes are detrimental to the care of patients is harder to document, but it is suspected. Patients have good reason to worry that conflict of interest situations for physicians lead to compromised care for patients.

Not all HMOs use incentives; those that put physicians on salary do not get into these particular problems. On the other hand, the lack of strong incentives is said to be the cause of some HMOs' financial failures. Doctors will worry about the financial health of the organization that pays their salary, and this also can cause conflict of interests. Third-party payer and financial incentive plans are complicated matters, but there are some assumptions underlying the debate about them that need to be brought to light.

1. Change is difficult and there is often a bias in favor of the status quo. So, in this debate, there seems to be an assumption that medicine-as-usual, private physician paid by individual patient, is free of conflict of interest and thus provides the best care.

What is forgotten is that in traditional practice there is a hidden incentive, one that is in fact the exact opposite of the one posed by cost-containment systems. On a fee-for-service system, physicians are rewarded for service; thus, the more check-ups, appointments, lab tests, surgical procedures they perform, the more they are rewarded. It is often a fine line in many cases between a test that is absolutely necessary and one that is advised "just to be on the safe side."

2. When individual physicians set their own standards and are responsible for all decisions, the tendency nowadays is to practice defensive medicine, which can be seen as an overutilization of resources, the prime goal of which is protection of the physician from legal suits. So, the trend toward limiting services imposed by HMOs can be seen as a cancelling out of some unnecessary and excessive services that physicians have been led into by fee-for-service practice.

Medicine as a Business

The trend toward HMOs and for-profit hospitals suggests a move from considering medicine a profession to considering it a business. What are the implications for health-care professionals if this happens? How will medicine change?

1. Medicine as a profession is self-regulating. Medical people decide who will get into medical school and how many, who gets licensed and board certified, what the professional standards of competence are, and who gets disciplined and loses the license to practice. Businesses, on the other hand, are regulated from the outside: by federal and state regulations and agencies. So if medicine becomes more like a business, one can expect control of the profession to change from internal to external.

2. Businesses are subject to a great many laws and regulations. As medicine becomes more like a business, even greater defensive medicine and its subsequent overutilization of resources may be expected.

3. The buyer–seller relationship is built on the principle of "Buyer beware." Although there are consumer protection regulations, it is a relationship built on formal contract, not on personal trust. This model will not work well for the doctor–patient relationship because patients generally cannot know enough about medical care to know when they are getting their money's worth and when they are not. From the physician's and nurse's point of view, it may rob medicine of some of its effectiveness and satisfactions, both of which depend on the trusting relationship with patients. If these changes are not attractive to those in the professions, then they must take steps to meet the demands for cost-efficient medicine without succumbing to the temptations to redesign it on the model of American business.

HMOs are beneficial because it is important to contain costs. However, physicians need to be aware of the problems and find an active role in the design and philosophy of health delivery systems to make them work in ways that will be both efficient and ethical.

Part V. Additional Cases for Discussion

1. A 9-year-old boy is recovering normally from an appendectomy. He is anxious to be discharged, but his parents would rather he stay another day or two "to be on the safe side." The doctor believes either decision would be medically justified, although he knows the hospital is pressing for earliest possible discharges.

    How much should he take into account the urging of the hospital?

2. An immigrant family refuses to consent to biopsy of a mass on their son's ear, because of cultural beliefs that his spirit will escape and cause great troubles. The attending pediatrician suggests a 1-week trial on antibiotics but the consultant is adamant about not altering the standard approach. "This could also be cancer," she states, and urges contacting the state child protection service.

    What reasons, if any, might justify "bending the rules?"

3. A 10-month-old infant is clinically deteriorating because of progressive biliary cirrhosis. The family desperately appeals to their pediatrician for aid in obtaining a liver transplant. "We need your assistance in a media campaign. And is there any possible candidate in the ICU that you could approach?"

    Should the doctor comply or advise the parents to go through the regional donor bank and "wait their turn"?

4. A young physician caring for a child recovering from an auto accident is having increasing difficulty dealing with the parents. They are suspicious, constantly question recommendations, and make excessive demands for services, explanations, and reassurances. Although the doctor likes and relates well with the child, he wonders if an older physician or one with a more authoritarian manner would manage the situation better. At any rate, he would be glad to be "rid of these disagreeable people."

    May the physician ethically withdraw from the case?

    What is the difference between withdrawing from and "abandoning" a patient?

5.   A parent asks a physician to take on the care of his child, who is acutely ill
with cough and fever, and is known to have AIDS. The child's previous
doctor is no longer available. The physician refuses, justifying this action as
within the acceptable limits of a "contractual view" of the doctor–patient
relationship.

Do doctors have special obligations to assume risk?

What are the limits of their responsibilities?

Part V. Suggested Reading

1. American Board of Pediatrics. Medical Ethics Subcommittee: Teaching and evaluation of interpersonal skills and ethical decision making in pediatrics. *Pediatrics*. 1987;79:829–833.
2. Groves JE. Taking care of the hateful patient. *N Engl J Med*. 1978;298:883–887.
3. Hoang SN, Erickson RV. Guidelines for providing medical care to Southeast Asian refugees. *JAMA*. 1982;248:710–714.
4. Kim JH, Perfect JR. To help the sick: an historical and ethical essay concerning the refusal to care for patients with AIDS. *Am J Med*. 1988;84:135–138.
5. MacIntyre A. The nature of virtues. *Hastings Center Report*. 1981;11(2):27–34.
6. May WF. Code, covenant, contract, or philanthropy. *Hastings Center Report*. 1975:5(6):26–38.
7. Morreim EH. Cost containment: challenging fidelity and justice. *Hastings Center Report*. 1988;18(6):20–25.
8. Nolan K, Bayer R, eds. AIDS: the responsibilities of health professionals. *Hastings Center Report*. 1988;18(2) (Special Suppl):1–32.
9. Paris JJ, Crone RK, Reardon F. Physician' refusal of requested treatment. The case of Baby L. *N Engl J Med*. 1990;322:1012–1015.
10. Wolf SM, ed. The persistent problem of PVS. *Hastings Center Report*. 1988;18(1):26–47.
11. Zuger A. Professional responsibilities in the AIDS generation. AIDS on the wards: a residency in medical ethics. *Hastings Center Report*. 1987;17(3):16–20.

Part VI
Treating Adolescents:
When Is a Child an Adult?

CHAPTER 21

Confidentiality

"Thanks for asking my Dad to step out for a minute. Can I talk to you about something? You're going to be doing a blood test for this virus I have, right? Do you suppose you could do an AIDS test at the same time? But I don't want you to say anything to my parents about it. You know me pretty well, right? I've been coming here for 16 years. I promise you, if the test is positive, I'll tell my Dad and Mom. But if it's negative, I don't want them to know anything about it. OK?"

"Rob, let me catch my breath for a second."

How much should the physician protect adolescent confidentiality?

Discussion Questions

1. What is the basis of parents' right to know?

2. What is the basis of adolescents' right to confidentiality?

3. Are there different obligations concerning confidentiality between a family pediatrician and one practicing in adolescent medicine?

This case epitomizes the dilemmas physicians face when treating adolescents who are, by definition, in the transitional period from childhood to full autonomy. Although the various states have granted full decision-making power with confidentiality to teenagers who need treatment for venereal disease, drug abuse, and so on, the justification has always been in terms of public health: if teens were not granted this immunity from parental knowledge, many of them would not come for treatment, thus continuing to endanger themselves and others through the spread of contagious disease or antisocial behavior.

When an individual teen is brought to the family physician or private pediatrician by parents, however, the situation seems different. There is little threat to public health, since the teen will be treated, if needed, either with or without the parents' knowledge.

The Basis of Rights

The conflict of obligation that the request for confidentiality generates raises interesting questions about the relationships among the three parties: the moral status of adolescent versus parents, the doctor–parent relationship, and the doctor–adolescent relationship.

1. **Adolescent–parent relationship**. Insofar as parents are normally the legal decision-makers for minor children, they need to be informed. Unless they waive the right to know, either explicitly by saying something like, "I don't need to know the details. Just go ahead and do what needs to be done and send me the bill," or implicitly by sending the teen to the physician by himself, it should be assumed that they want to know and have a presumed right to know.

A more practical concern is that in serious situations, the adolescent will need both the financial and emotional support of his family. It is difficult to imagine an adolescent dealing on his own with infectious mononucleosis or colitis, much less AIDS. In Rob's case, however, the adolescent is not proposing to keep an AIDS diagnosis confidential, but only the fact that he may have been exposed to AIDS. What he proposes dealing with on his own is his anxiety about AIDS, not the disease itself. The practical reasons for involving family, then, are not so great.

This leads to the straightforward moral question: Do parents have the right to know? It might be helpful to consider a position on adolescent confidentiality in contexts other than medicine. Do parents have the right to know school grades and the results of standardized tests? Most would agree that they do. Do parents have the right to information that would be on tax forms, that is, how many hours the teen has worked and how much pay he has received? Probably yes. Do parents have the right to know where the teen is at night, who his friends are, what he keeps in his bureau drawer?

Those who defend the right of parents to know might base their reasons on the kind of argument Locke gives about the source of parental authority: parents have the right to limit the liberty of children because they have a duty to society to bring up the child and educate him in a certain way, and in order to fulfill their duty it is necessary to have authority over him. Thus, confidentiality may be breached by parents when it is necessary to ensure the safety and welfare of the child. Locke also suggests, however, that the goal of parental guardianship is to nurture the rational and autonomous powers of children, so that they may be free of parental supervision at adulthood. This implies an inverse relationship between increasing maturity and parental obligation and supervision.

This analysis suggests a guideline for confidentiality between parent and child. The younger and less mature the child, the greater the right of the parent to know; the more mature the child, that is, the less likely that respecting confidentiality may harm him, the lesser the right of the parent to know. If the physician applies this principle, he decides whether or not to respect the adolescent's confidentiality depending on whether or not he sees it as a threat to the well-being of the child. If he trusts that Rob will confide in his parents if the AIDS test is positive, or if he tells Rob that he, the doctor, will break confidentiality if Rob does not, then he may judge that the parents' right to know is diminished because keeping confidentiality will not put Rob at risk of harm. If

Rob had asked for confidentiality even in the face of a positive test result, then the calculation of risk of harm would be different.

2. **The physician–parent relationship.** There are two basic options: to view oneself as primarily the parents' ally or primarily as the adolescent's ally. Being a parents' ally implies a "tell everything" position, with no regard for the evolving maturity of the adolescent. It runs the risk of resulting in lack of candor on the part of the adolescent, thus compromising his medical care. Moreover, it ignores the duty of the physician to care for the psychological and emotional needs of the patient as well as the organic needs. To be wholly the adolescent's ally and give too-easy agreement to keep confidentiality in all circumstances is not consistent with the welfare of the adolescent and violates the right of the parents, based on their need to know in order to carry out their role as decision-makers.

A middle of the road position that is honest to both parties is something like this: "I won't tell your parents, but you have to promise to tell them," or, in the case of IV drug abuse, "go for counseling." Or: "I won't tell your parents, but I will help you to tell them if you want me to," or "I intend to keep trying to persuade you until you do."

3. **The doctor–adolescent relationship.** As we have seen, the utilitarian argument for confidentiality that is successful in the public health arena is not relevant in the case where the adolescent is brought in by parents. The question at issue is not treatment versus nontreatment but treatment either with or without confidentiality. Thus, a different kind of argument is often used, which assumes that the parents want whatever is in the best interest of their son, assumes that they would gladly consent to appropriate treatment if asked, and that they will thank you afterward. The thank-you argument is a way of trying to justify paternalism. If the person for whom the decision is made is later grateful, this signals implicit consent—retroactively, as it were. It is not a terribly strong argument, but if used in these situations, it allows physicians to view themselves as acting in loco parentis, thus strengthening the relationship between adolescent and physician.

On the other hand, these rights are not unconditional. Factors to consider include the seriousness of the medical situation, the maturity of the adolescent, and the predicted effect on the parent-child relationship. In Rob's case, the medical situation is obviously serious if the test is positive. Even if the test is negative, Rob is in serious trouble if he is continuing whatever behavior put him at risk for AIDS. On the other hand, his proposal to request confidentiality about the testing but not about a positive test result suggests a reasonably high level of maturity. Finally, the physician's knowledge of the family and his belief that Rob's father will not be overly punitive if he discovers the lack of complete openness will also need to be considered.

A final question might be raised: Is keeping confidentiality, which in this case amounts to withholding information, the same as deception or lying? Contrast Rob's particular request for confidentiality with a different request that he might have made: if the test result is positive, of course I'll tell my parents, but could you tell them it was caused by that transfusion I had when I had my tonsils out? The physician should not agree to this kind of proposal. Yet, to encourage teens to seek out treatment, physicians may sometimes rely on vague terms, such as "Your daughter has "pelvic inflammation" instead of saying, "Your daughter has VD." Parents who do not pursue further explanations may be choosing not to know more or may be already so far removed from their children's lives that confidentiality is appropriate.

The Adolescent Specialist

In the case described, the parent is already involved, both by the fact of having brought his son to the physician and by the fact that the physician has had an ongoing relationship with the family. Prima facie, at least, it seems that the physician has an obligation both to parent and child. By contrast, a physician in an adolescent clinic where teens may come by themselves has a relationship and thus an obligation primarily or perhaps exclusively with the adolescent patient.

In contrast to pediatricians or family doctors, those who specialize in adolescent medicine, it seems, have a different "contract" with their patients. Parents are more legitimately out of the picture, although they may continue to pay the bills, and the physician must give primary concern to what is good for the adolescent. When issues of confidentiality arise, they should be resolved in the same way issues of confidentiality might be handled in adult medicine. If a wife requests that information be withheld from husband or children, that should be respected, unless there is specific risk to other individuals. If the physician is convinced this would not be to the welfare of the patient, then she must use persuasion and negotiation.

The pediatrician who continues to see children through their teens can often find a way to mark the transition from child to adult by saying to the parents something like this: "Now that Rob is 13, I'd like to have a chance to talk with him alone." Although the teen may never use the opportunity to confide anything he does not want his parents to know, it provides a way to do so if he wishes, and sends the message to the parents that this is the time to begin to respect confidentiality. The important thing is to be clear to both parent and adolescent that there are some things that should be between teen and doctor only, but that confidentiality is not absolute; it is conditional and depends on the physician's judgment of the risk of serious harm that it might incur.

CHAPTER 22

Legal Issues

"Dr. Carey, I really need some help. My parents don't know this, but I've been going around with a bunch of kids a lot older than I am. Everyone thinks I'm 17, even though I'm only 14. But I'm in over my head now with this boy. I think I need to talk to a professional counselor, but my parents don't believe in that sort of thing and my school doesn't have anyone. I could pay for it out of my summer earnings—that wouldn't be a problem. Can you suggest someone and arrange it for me? And, in the meantime, could you give me a prescription for birth control pills? Is it legal for me to get them, and without my parents knowing?"

"You're asking a lot of questions, Sue. Let's take them one at a time."

What are the legal and moral limits on treatment of adolescents without parental consent?

Discussion Questions

1. Since Sue can pay her own medical expenses, is she an emancipated minor?

2. What are the legal limits and obligations of the pediatrician to adolescents and their parents?

3. What are the pediatrician's moral obligations to adolescent patients and their parents?

Adolescence as we know it is a fairly recent phenomenon and in a sense our society has not really resolved its ambivalence about how adolescents should be treated. In some contexts they are given rights and responsibilities in recognition of their status as near-adults, yet in other contexts they are protected and restricted in the same way as younger children. In order to guide professionals as well as to assign status to adolescents and in some cases to protect the public, legislators have developed a whole body of specific laws regulating the medical treatment of this age group. The laws vary from state to state; some are age-based and some call for physicians' judgment. In any case, all pediatricians need to be aware of the regulations that apply to their particular practice.

First and foremost, it must be noted that even the most comprehensive knowledge of state and federal laws and policies cannot answer every question, and even the most vigorous adherence to the letter and spirit of the law cannot completely protect a physician or hospital against possible lawsuits or charges of malpractice. The way the legal system operates, virtually anyone can bring charges against anyone else. Indeed, pediatricians are especially vulnerable. The statute of limitations that sets a limit on the length of time within which a person can bring a lawsuit applies in medical cases only after the time of "discovery," that is, when the damage is discovered, not when the event or alleged malpractice occurred. For children, the statute of limitations is extended so that it begins only after they have reached the age of 18. Thus, in theory at least, a case can be brought by or for a child at almost any time.

Yet, despite its potential for misuse, the very vagueness of law is its strength, and physicians should recognize it as such. It is the absence or vagueness of law that allows physicians to work within an ethical framework and to individualize medical care. This is especially important in the care of adolescents, where the variation in maturity is great even within the same chronological age group.

The alternative to the present vagueness of law would be a system of strict regulation, with every decision subject to guidelines and age standardization. This might afford the medical profession some guarantee against suit and afford patients protection against a physician's evil intentions or bad judgment, but even if it were possible to accomplish, it would leave no room for discretion or judgment. One must then recognize that physicians have to take responsibility for what they do and must live with a less than perfect sense of security. Practicing medicine well and developing honest and trusting relationships with patients are good ways to practice "defensive" medicine.

Emancipated Minors

Included in the body of law that is available to guide practice with adolescents is the special legal category of emancipated minor. It is recognized by 34 states and allows accommodation to the needs of adolescents in different stages of maturity and with varying degrees of closeness or dependence on parents and guardians. Generally, an emancipated minor is someone younger than 18 years, who is not living at home and/or is self-supporting, married, in military service, an unmarried mother, or whose parents have agreed to emancipation. Such an adolescent may consent to medical treatment without parental consent or knowledge. College students, although not strictly fulfilling these conditions, may also be considered emancipated for the purpose of giving medical consent, but boarding school students may not. An unmarried teenage mother may consent for treatment of her child (although in some localities she is not able to consent for herself!)

When Sue asks for a referral for counseling, she is not really asking for treatment, but it is still appropriate to determine if she is an emancipated minor. Clearly, she is not. Are there, however, other recognized criteria according to which she could be allowed to consent for herself?

In addition to providing for emancipation of minors, a few states have created statutes, and virtually all states acknowledge under common law the status of mature minor. This allows physicians to treat with only the minor's consent, if (1) in the physician's judgment the minor is able to understand the procedure and its risks sufficiently to give informed consent, (2) the treatment is for the minor's own benefit, (3) the treatment is considered less than major or serious, (4) it is considered necessary by conservative medical opinion, and (5) there is reason, including simply the minor's request, why parental consent cannot be obtained. The physician should further determine the patient's competency, under the usual adult standards, and obtain informed consent. It is reassuring to know that there are no reported cases in which a physician has been found liable for treating a minor age 15 years or over when these conditions have been met.

Applying these criteria to Sue, the physician might note on the side of her maturity the fact that she has found opportunity to confide her concerns and has at least thought about the question of payment. However, the fact that she is only 14 is a prima facie reason against considering her a mature minor, and whether or not she was accompanied by her mother might also be considered.

Legal Limits and Moral Obligations

On the question about birth control measures, the legal issue is somewhat easier. Virtually all states allow minors to consent for their own treatment for reproductive concerns, venereal disease, and drug and alcohol abuse.

Suppose the pediatrician concludes that it is legally permissible to give Sue a confidential referral for counseling and prescribe birth control measures for her. However, since Sue is neither emancipated nor a mature minor, the doctor is not legally required to do so. There is still room, then, to ask, What are the physician's moral obligations to both parents and adolescents?

Many moral issues about decision-making remain open, even after the legal issues are clear. Thus, every pediatrician must develop a certain "style" of dealing with adolescents and their parents, a way of responding to their needs and claims that reflects the ethical parameters within which he or she will practice. If one of the major challenges for pediatricians is to help adolescents grow up and take on responsibility for their own health care, then they must think out guidelines for appropriate sharing of decision-making among teenagers, parents, and physician. In their interaction with adolescents, physicians can serve as models for parents to learn how to "let go." The physician's respect and encouragement of the young teenager's developing maturity allows the parents to see their child in a new light. It also enhances the adolescent's perception of herself.

Letting go can be hard for the pediatrician as well. Patients who first present as adolescents are easy to relate to as adolescents, but it may be more difficult to effect the changes in the doctor–patient relationship required by the emerging teen whom one has known since birth. One must make subtle but deliberate alterations in approach in order not to lose the opportunity for teenagers to perceive the physician as a resource for information and counseling as they wean themselves from total dependence on parents.

As contrasted to the clearly symbiotic relationship between young children and parents, teens and parents are involved in a relationship that requires delicate and responsible balancing between the needs of the teen for continuing family support and protection and their need for increasing exercise of independence. Quite apart from the claims of parents to the right to consent and to know, argument can be made for not following the wishes of the teenager. Treatment in the area of mental health, for example, should usually not be kept confidential from parents because parents cannot help and protect the child without information. Furthermore, treatment is less likely to be successful if the whole family is not involved. Similar arguments can be made against confidentiality in treating a very young pregnant teenager: although disclosure will be painful, the gain may be worth it in those cases where she would benefit from the counsel and practical help of her family.

Even if one accepts this line of reasoning, there are different ways for the physician to play intermediary between teen and parent. Many times the ideal way is to persuade the young teen to confide in her parents herself or for the physician to volunteer to discuss it with them on her behalf. On the other hand, argument can be made for complying with the wishes of teenagers against parental involvement. In certain cases it may be clear in the physician's judgment that the consequences of involving the parents may not be beneficial and in fact may be harmful to the adolescent. Or, the physician may recognize this adolescent as being a truly mature minor and thus should respect her right of self-determination. This does not, however, preclude giving advice and making recommendations.

CHAPTER 23

Teenage Suicide

"I had two cases today that really troubled me."

"You look pretty down. Tell me about them."

"I saw the first this morning at clinic. Renee is only 15 and recovering from her fourth suicide attempt in the past 2 years. She has a horrible home life, is under the care of the state, and has been referred to a residential treatment home, but there is a 4 to 6-month wait. I wonder what will happen to her. Then in the afternoon at my office I saw Sam, a 13-year-old boy. His mother began by complaining about his 'acting out' behavior and mentioned that he had dropped out of his baseball team at school. The kid appeared in good health, but sullen and unresponsive. All he said the whole time was, 'What difference does it make, anyway?'"

"So, you're worried that the 13-year-old will turn out to be suicidal like the 15-year-old. But what can you do about it?"

How should the medical profession think about adolescent suicide?

Discussion Questions

1. Is there such a thing as rational suicide? If so, can it apply to adolescents?

2. What are the pediatrician's responsibilities to suicidal teens? to society?

Statistics show that suicide is currently the third leading cause of death among adolescents and accounts for 12% of the mortality among adolescents and young adults. It is estimated that 4% of all high school students have made suicide attempts within the past year. The true extent of suicidal behavior is not really known, since studies have shown that as few as 12% come to medical attention. Medical students or residents are called upon to treat such cases in the emergency room and private pediatricians care for children and adolescents who are at risk for self-inflicted harm. Thus, the responsibility for being knowledgeable and helpful about the medical, social, and psychological aspects of prevention and treatment are very great.

There seem to be three levels of potential suicide. The most obvious is the consciously planned suicide attempt, as in swallowing a bottle of aspirin or shutting oneself in the garage with the car motor running. At the second level, there is suicidal ideation: the individual thinks about suicide, drops verbal hints about having nothing to live for, draws away emotionally from others, but takes no overt action to implement a plan. There is evidence that this kind of thinking can be "contagious" in some peer groups. At the third level, there is what might be called suicidal behavior, for example, drinking and driving at high speeds. If asked whether or not they intended to kill themselves, the now-sober drivers would say, "Of course not." But they clearly know the risks and seem to be tempting fate, albeit unconsciously.

There are different assumptions about the nature of suicide attempts, and they give rise to different conclusions about the ethical responsibilities and limits of the physician in responding to potential suicides. Applying these assumptions to adolescents as always presents special problems. There is a constant tension between the ethical imperative to respect their growing ability to make choices for themselves and responsibility to protect them from serious harm. One common assumption made about all unsuccessful suicide attempts is that they are cries for help. Recent studies suggest that about two thirds of adolescent suicide attempts are for reasons other than a desire to die. If this view is adopted, then it might seem quite reasonable to treat the adolescent who has attempted suicide as a child in need and thus adopt a quite frankly paternalistic stance toward her, at the expense of her desire and need for self-determination.

Suicide and Rationality

Another common assumption is that no one who attempts to end his or her own life can be entirely rational. The kind of depression that leads to suicide attempts is a serious psychological handicap, it is said, and therefore the attempted suicide should always be considered noncompetent. Again, a strongly paternalistic stance seems justified. The same reasoning would apply to an adolescent and an adult alike, justifying a denial of autonomy in either case.

On the other hand, there is a real question about the validity of these assumptions. Are they assuming what needs to be proven? What evidence is there, apart from the suicide attempt itself, that all suicide attempts are thinly disguised calls for help or that all suicide attempts are the result of irrational thinking? Thus, the question must be asked: Can a suicide ever be rational? Can a life be so full of suffering and pain that one is justified in ending it? If so, then do others have an obligation not to interfere?

Leaving aside for the moment the special issues about adolescence, what would be the necessary conditions of a rational suicide? First, a rational suicide can be committed only by a rational person. This includes having the ability to reason, having adequate information, and having a realistic world-view. Those whose rationality is impaired, say by depression, may fail to see possible alternatives and may not have a realistic idea of their own place in the world, perhaps because of very low self-esteem, paranoia, or an overly inflated ego. Second, rational persons will try to avoid harm and pain. Thus, in order for a suicide to be considered rational, it must be judged as the best and only alternative to a life of virtually nothing but pain and harm. This judgment must be based on correct and adequate information about the self and the world, present and future.

Thus, if a competent reasoning person with adequate information and a realistic world-view judges his or her own life to be not worth living in terms of pain and harm, then that person's suicide may be considered rational. Given these conditions, one may then invoke Mill's principle that the only legitimate reason for interfering with the actions of rational adults is for the good of society. Interfering in something that affects only the person who is acting is never justified. Unless there is some overriding social reason for a person who is adult and rational not to commit suicide, the appropriate ethical response would seem to be respect for that person's self-determination and nonintervention.

If rational suicide is based on judgments of pain and harm, then there is little if any difference between rational suicide and voluntary euthanasia. One possible difference is that the term "euthanasia" is generally applied to cases where there is physical suffering, whereas the term "suicide" is more often applied when there is mental suffering. If in addition it is assumed that mental pain compromises rationality, whereas physical pain does not necessarily do so, then it is understandable why euthanasia is often considered morally acceptable but suicide is not. However, it was argued above that the assumption that mental pain impairs rationality cannot be made without empirical evidence. One should not be able to rule out the possibility of rational suicide simply by definition.

Granting, then, that a rational suicide is possible, can it apply to adolescents? Can the criteria be met by someone who is not a rational adult? In one sense, of course, the answer has to be no, for an adolescent is not an adult. On the criterion of being a rational person, however, an adolescent could qualify, for it has been shown (see Chapter 2) that there is little difference between the reasoning of 14 year olds and 18 or 21 year olds, especially concerning medical treatment decisions. Now, suicide is not a medical treatment decision, but perhaps it is close enough. The point is that if Mill's principle is a good reason to respect the rights of rational, informed adults to suicide, there is at least prima facie reason to extend the same right to rational adolescents. In practical terms, however, it is almost impossible to imagine a case where a pediatrician should stand by and do nothing about a potential adolescent suicide. After all, they are minors, and suicide if successful is an irreversible action.

The younger the person the more likely it is that circumstances can be improved and the pain of one's life diminished. One would hope that, even in as difficult a case as Renee's, when society has not provided the resources to care for her properly, there can be some change for the better. Suicide attempts like Renee's end up at the doorstep of the pediatrician because of medical need, and insofar as the pediatrician is the advocate of the whole child, not just her physical being, there is a responsibility to know of the available community resources, and if resources are not available, the pediatrician should be an outspoken advocate for their development.

Protection versus Privacy

The doctor's frustration with Renee's situation leads her to think more in terms of suicide prevention. Could someone have intervened at an earlier stage in her history? Was Renee at one time giving out the same kinds of signals as Sam is now giving? Is Sam's difficult behavior and negative comment a sign of potential self-destructive behavior or just an expression of typical teenage attitudes?

It is typical and normal for adolescents to exhibit emotional turmoil, some suicidal ideation, an intense need for privacy, and a drive to practice self-determination. All of these must find expression in the teenager's life but any of them could be mistaken for signs of serious trouble. The pediatrician may need to probe areas that adolescents would rather keep private and intervene where they want to keep control.

There is an obvious tension between respecting privacy and protecting life. The obligation to protect takes precedence and this is a case where one should err on the side of caution.

These issues underline again the critical nature of doctor–patient relationships with adolescents. The pediatrician who knows a child well can better determine what is normal development for that child. If the physician has known Sam over a long period of time, she can reassure his mother by reminding her how willful he was as a 3-year-old, so it is no surprise that he is balking at school and parental authority and organized sports at 13. For those adolescents who are not known to the pediatrician, a good medical history is imperative, with plenty of opportunity for questions about activities, attitudes, and possible emotional problems.

CHAPTER 24

Changing a Lifestyle

"You can go home tomorrow, Ted. But we need to talk first. You've not been taking care of yourself."

"Yeah, I know. You can skip the lectures. I know all about my diabetes and all the things I'm not supposed to eat and drink. Especially drink."

"Yes. This is the second time you've landed in the hospital on a Saturday night. Drinking like that isn't so good for anyone, but for you, it can be really dangerous. Your blood sugar drops out of sight! That can lead to permanent brain damage."

"I'm sorry, Doc. But it's my life. I want to be like everyone else and when they drink beer, I'm going to drink beer. So, sometimes we go over the limit."

What are the physician's responsibilities to adolescents with unhealthy life styles?

Discussion Questions

1. What should be the role of parents?

2. What are the ethical limits of persuasion?

3. When, if ever, may one "give up" on a patient?

If Ted were an adult, the limits of what his physician could and should do about getting him to change his life style would be fairly clear. Despite "doctor's orders," all the physician can really do is offer advice. It is the role of physicians in dealing with adults, to educate patients about their condition, present the facts and be sure the patient understands, and do their best to get patients to recognize that following medical advice is in their own best interest. Physicians ought to use persuasion and the authority of their expertise to make the case compelling and offer help and support, but after that patients are expected to assume responsibility for their own adult behavior. They must be the ones to choose to change or not. Coercion is not an option and the role of nagging nurse-maid is inappropriate.

However, because Ted is not an adult, the question of the limits of the physician's obligations and the methods that may be used in securing the patient's best interest are open to debate. Perhaps the role of nagging nursemaid is appropriate when counseling is not effective. Furthermore, the problem Ted's physician faces is not merely noncompliance; he must convince his patient to begin to change his whole life style. This is, as we know, a difficult thing for anyone to do. For the adolescent who is striving for independence from adults and is especially anxious to fit in with his peers, committing himself to a different life style, even for reasons of his own good health, is extremely difficult.

The Role of Parents

The most natural place to turn for help in convincing Ted to change is to his parents. The pattern throughout childhood is that the physician advises parents on medical treatment and they see to it that it is carried out. They administer the pills, keep the child in bed or out of school, eliminate certain things from his diet, convince, cajole, or intimidate him into compliance. Clearly none of these things will work in the same way any more once the child reaches adolescence. Nor should they. Rather, the goal of both physician and parent should be to educate the child and gradually initiate him into taking responsibility for his own health.

Apart from the ineffectiveness and inappropriateness of turning the problem over to Ted's parents, there is the question of threatening the delicate balance of the doctor–patient relationship. Strict duties of confidentiality are not due to an adolescent, and the treatment of diabetes does not warrant the concern about confidentiality that the treatment of VD would. Still, Ted's drinking is probably already an issue of contention between parents and teen, so the physician can show respect for Ted's status as no longer a mere child by dealing with him directly and not through his parents.

On the other hand, if Ted has demonstrated that he is not especially mature for his age, if his behavior is more like a 13-year-old than a 17-year-old, if he is living at home and generally defers to his parents for advice and care, then it might be quite acceptable to treat him like a younger child and involve his parents more directly in trying to persuade or even to monitor his drinking.

Persuasion

The first line of attack should be persuasion. There are different kinds and different levels of persuasion, however, each with different ethical impact.

1. **Rational persuasion.** One view of the best of all possible worlds is that all persons, even teenagers, would be completely rational. This would involve these things: (1) being able to understand information, (2) being able to recognize good reasons for doing something, and (3) being able to conform behavior to good reasons. This view also assumes that all rational persons have some degree of self-interest. Thus, if it can be shown that doing x will contribute to their own

well-being and that doing y will be against their self-interest, they will unfailingly choose x over y.

There are metaphysical assumptions lurking beneath this analysis. The central one is an assumption of free will. Frequently misunderstood, free will does not imply acting free of causality, but rather acting from one's own good reasons, that is, from internal motivation. To be unfree is to be compelled to act by outside forces. Thus, on this view, to persuade someone to change his life style one would have to provide a clear account of the cause and effect relationship between actions of certain kinds—in Ted's case, drinking too much—and results that violate his self-interest—his immediate danger of injury and long-term damage to his health.

The advantage to rational persuasion is that it demonstrates respect for persons. It assumes that individuals have self-respect and want the best for themselves and are in control of their own lives.

2. **Nonrational persuasion.** Many forms of psychological theory adopt a form of determinism, which explains human behavior in terms of external causality. The extreme forms of this are recognized as addictions, compulsions, or neuroses where subjects may consciously want to change their behavior but cannot do so. This explains the mechanism of behavior modification programs, which create new sets of cause–effect relationships, resulting in altered behavior.

Subscribing to a simple deterministic model of human behavior that does not take into account a rational, conscious component may leave the door open for nonrational, ethically suspect methods of persuasion. One can get children and probably adolescents to change behavior by manipulation, deception, or coercion. One could also argue that the end justifies the means: that any method that works is acceptable because it is so important that Ted stop his self-destructive behavior. Needless to say, this is not a position to be recommended.

Giving Up

Responses that may be appropriate for noncompliant adult patients are not necessarily appropriate for adolescents. At some point it may be right for a physician to say to an adult, "I can't keep treating you if you don't comply. Perhaps someone else may have better success."

There is a stronger responsibility to "stand by" the adolescent who is suffering from his own life style. Relationships with adults may be harder for him to establish at that age and psychological abandonment more of a threat. Thus, those who already play the role of responsible adults in the teen's life need to take that responsibility very seriously. Until he is truly adult, Ted should not be left to the consequences of his own folly. The teenager must always be presented with hope for change.

Part VI. Additional Cases for Discussion

1. A 15-year-old boy is having a check-up required for participation in his high school's football program. He is accompanied by his father who privately asks the physician to screen his son's urine for anabolic steroids. "His temper is so short these days, and his muscles are just exploding. What's more, I think a lot of the kids are using these drugs, and I bet the coach knows it!"

    Should the physician comply with the father's request?

    If the urine test is positive, should he contact the high school?

    Assume the school requested the physician to develop a drug screening program as a prerequisite to athletic participation. Should the physician cooperate?

2. A 14-year-old girl is brought to her physician by her mother for recurrent vomiting over the last few weeks. On seeing the teenager alone, he learns that she is sexually active, and a pregnancy test proves positive. She says, "I thought this might be the problem. I know where to get an abortion. Please tell my Mom that it's just a viral infection!"

    How should the physician respond?

    If the test were negative, then what ought to be done?

3. A beauty-conscious mother brings her 13-year-old daughter to a plastic surgeon because of the child's large nose. The child is reluctant to have the operation.

    Is the mother's consent sufficient for the surgery?

    If the teenager wanted the operation and the mother objected, would the 13-year-old's consent be sufficient?

4. A 17-year-old hemophiliac admits to being sexually active with his girlfriend but refuses to be tested for HIV infection, despite his parents' urging and physician's recommendation. Furthermore, he demands that no one contact his girlfriend concerning his hemophilia or risk of AIDS.

Are there sufficient grounds for overriding the teenager's right to privacy?

Part VI. Suggested Reading

1. American Academy of Pediatrics, Committee on Adolescence, Committee on Bioethics, and Provisional Committee on Substance Abuse. Screening for drugs of abuse in children and adolescents. *Pediatrics.* 1989;84:396–398.
2. Brent DA. Suicide.and suicidal behavior in children and adolescents. *Pediatr Rev.* 1989;10:269–275.
3. Buchanan AE, Brock D. Chapter 5: Minors, I. Noninfant minors. In: *Deciding for Others. The Ethics of Surrogate Decision Making.* Cambridge: Cambridge University Press; 1989:216–246.
4. Halligan JB, Halligan LF, Snyder MB. Anabolic-androgenic steroid use by athletes. *N Engl J Med.* 1989;321:1042–1045.
5. Holder AR: Minors' rights to consent to medical care. *JAMA.* 1987;257:3400–3402.

Bibliography

Anthologies

1. Arras J, Rhoden N, eds. *Ethical Issues in Modern Medicine*, 3rd ed. Mountain View, Calif: Mayfield Publishing Co; 1989.
2. Beauchamp TL, Walters L, eds. *Contemporary Issues in Bioethics*, 3rd ed. Belmont, Calif: Wadsworth Publishing Co; 1989.
3. Gorovitz S, Macklin R, Jameton AL, O'Connor JM, Sherwin S, eds. *Moral Problems in Medicine*, 2nd ed. Englewood Cliffs, NJ: Prentice-Hall, Inc; 1983.
4. Mappes TA, Zembaty JS, eds. *Biomedical Ethics*, 3rd ed. NY: McGraw-Hill; 1991.

General Works

1. Beauchamp TL, Childress JF. *Principles of Biomedical Ethics*, 3rd ed. Oxford: Oxford University Press; 1989.
2. Munson R. *Intervention and Reflection–Basic Issues in Medical Ethics*, 3rd ed. Belmont, Calif: Wadsworth Publishing Co; 1988.
3. Reich WT, ed. *Encyclopedia of Bioethics*. Vols 1–4. New York: The Free Press; 1978.

Pediatrics

1. Coulter DL, Murray TH, Cerreto MC. Practical ethics in pediatrics. *Curr Probl Pediatr*. March, 1988:137–195.
2. Jonsen AR. The ethics of pediatric medicine. In Rudolph AM, ed. *Pediatrics*, 18th ed. Conn: Appleton & Lange; 1987:9-16.
3. Kopelman LM, Moskop JC. *Children and Health Care—Moral and Social Issues*. Dordrecht, The Netherlands: Kluwer Academic Publishers; 1989.
4. Marsh FH. *The Emerging Rights of Children in Treatment for Mental and Catastrophic Illnesses*. Washington, DC: University Press of America; 1979.
5. Silber T, ed. *Ethical Issues in the Treatment of Children and Adolescents*. Thorofare, NJ: Slack; 1983.
6. Truman JT, Van Eys J, Pochedly C, eds. *Human Values in Pediatric Hematology/Oncology*. NY: Praeger Publishers; 1986.
7. Weil WB: Ethical issues in pediatrics. *Curr Probl Pediatr*. Dec, 1989:619–665.

Glossary

Abandonment of patient

Termination of a doctor–patient relationship by a physician without reasonable notice or adequately arranging for continuation of needed care.

Active vs. passive euthanasia

See Euthanasia.

Advance directives

Instructions by a competent individual for future health care if incompetency should develop. Examples include a Living will and Durable power of attorney for health care.

Age-specific values

Values that are typically held by persons of a certain age, e.g., by teenagers, or given high priority during that time.

Assent

Agreement to research or treatment, given by a child or minor not old enough to give legally valid informed consent.

Autonomy

The ability and/or right to be self-determining; to be able to choose for oneself.

"Baby Doe" regulations

Federal regulations (1985) concerning principles of treatment of seriously handicapped newborns; in particular, that withholding "medically indicated" treatment from such infants is a form of child abuse and neglect, and that such action will cause states to lose federal grants for child abuse programs.

Benefit/burden ratio

See Risk/benefit analysis.

Benevolent deception
Lying or deception for the benefit of the person deceived.

Closed awareness
Knowing, e.g., a diagnosis, where each party who knows also knows that the others know but no one talks about it.

Competent
Legally recognized to be able to make decisions for oneself; minors are presumed to be incompetent, except under certain specified conditions, which vary from state to state.

Conscience
A personal sense, generally intuitive and urgent, of what one ought to do or not do. Often described, as by Socrates, as an inner voice that forbids certain actions.

Contract model, contractual arrangement
(1) A formal arrangement between individuals, usually a document that delineates the specific duties/responsibilities/obligations and their limits for each party. (2) A view of the doctor–patient relationship as a formal arrangement that delineates specific obligations and limits for each party. (contrast with Covenant model)

Cost/benefit analysis
See Risk/benefit analysis.

Covenant model
A view of the doctor–patient relationship as a solemn mutual agreement involving trust and fidelity. Contrasted with the Contract model, it is an open-ended and growing relationship.

DNR, do not resuscitate
Medical orders that, should a patient develop a cardiopulmonary arrest, no attempts at resuscitation should be undertaken, i.e., "No Code" orders.

Double effect, principle of	A moral argument used to defend certain actions that can be anticipated to have both good and bad outcomes such an act is claimed to be acceptable if: (1) it is in itself not bad, (2) it is intended to cause the good effect, (3) the evil outcome is not the means to the good one, and (4) the overall outcome is favorably balanced. For example, in a dying patient, giving a dose of narcotic necessary to control pain, knowing (but not intending) that it might hasten death.
Durable power of attorney for health care	A form of advance directive in which a person specifies who should make health decisions if the person has become incompetent.
Emancipated minor	A teenaged minor who is free of parental control for giving informed consent to any medical treatment; based on legal statutes that vary among states but use relatively objective criteria, such as marriage, pregnancy, or parenthood, living independently, military service, high school graduation, or whose parents have surrendered their parental rights. (compare with Mature minor)
Euthanasia	Literally a good death; hastening death to alleviate suffering.
Active (or positive)	Taking a positive action, e.g., giving an overdose of a narcotic.
Passive (or negative)	Withholding or withdrawing life supports, e.g., not ordering antibiotics for an infection. It is a matter of debate whether there is a moral distinction between these kinds of actions.
Voluntary	Requested by competent patients for themselves.
Involuntary	Decided by others, generally in situations in which the patient is judged incompetent.
Futile treatment	Treatment which will not achieve the intended goal.

Informed consent	Permission given by patient or proxy for purposes of treatment or research; can be given only by competent adult who is sufficiently informed and uncoerced.
Just distribution	Fair distribution of benefits and burdens in a society.
Living will	A form of advance directive in which a person specifies what kinds of treatments are desired for different medical conditions, should the person be incompetent to decide.
Mature minor	A teenaged minor who may give consent because the physician judges that he or she understands the nature, purposes, and risks of the proposed treatment; generally limited to minors at least 15 years old where the treatment is for the patient's own benefit and is judged necessary by conservative medical opinion. (compare with Emancipated minor)
ORM (orders for resuscitative measures)	Medical orders specifying the resuscitative measures to be employed for different types of cardiorespiratory failure in a given patient.
Paternalism	Imposing a decision on another person for that person's welfare; the theory that "doctor knows best."
Persistent vegetative state	A state of total lack of awareness, which has continued for several weeks with virtually no likelihood of recovery. Brain-stem components of the nervous system and vegetative functions are operative, associated with absence of cognitive and cerebral cortex processing. Not brain dead or simply in coma.
Pluralistic	Nonhomogeneous; refers to a society that includes different ethnic, religious, cultural, or racial groups.
Practical reasoning	Reasoning that results in or is intended to result in action; not just theoretical.
Prima facie	Literally, on the face of it, at first view; refers to rights or duties that can be overridden by more stringent rights or duties.

Principle of double effect   See Double effect, principle of..

Principle of utility   See utilitarianism, utilitarian reasoning

Protectionism   The view that protecting children is more important than giving them liberties.

Proxy consent   Consent for treatment or research, given by a parent or guardian, for a child or an incompetent adult.

Randomized clinical trials   A research method for determining optimal therapy among different treatments patients are assigned by random selection to the therapies being compared; as in standard versus experimental treatment.

Reasonable person standard   A kind of proxy consent, choosing for another as a reasonable person would; applicable when the special interests and values of the person are not known, as with an infant. (contrast with Subjective standard)

Rehearsal in the imagination   Thinking through a hypothetical situation in order to be prepared for decision-making in actual situations.

Rights   Moral or legal claims by one party against another.

Risk/benefit analysis   A method of choosing the best treatment by identifying and weighing, in terms of probabilities of occurrence and magnitude of effect, the possible risks (of harm) and benefits of the available options. also referred to as Benefit/burden ratio, Cost/benefit analysis or Harm/benefit analysis.

Shared decision-making   Patient or proxyand physician participate together in coming to a treatment decision.

Slippery slope argument

(1) A type of argument that warns against taking a certain action, which in itself may seem right because there will be an inevitable progression to a wrong action. (2) The presumption is that there are no rational or socially effective distinctions (stopping points) between the two actions, and thus taking the first will place one on a slippery slope toward the second. Also called the wedge argument. A common example allowing voluntary euthanasia will lead to acceptance of involuntary euthanasia.

Standard therapy

Therapy generally employed by the medical profession, based on demonstrated validity or historical precedent as opposed to nonstandard therapy used by one or more physicians in experimental and/or desperate situations.

Subjective standard

A kind of proxy consent; choosing for another as that person would have chosen, according to that person's values. (contrast with Reasonable person standard)

Substituted judgment

See Subjective standard.

Supererogatory

Above and beyond the call of duty.

Therapeutic vs. nontherapeutic research

Therapeutic research has as its primary goals both the patient's welfare and the generation of new information; nontherapeutic research aims only for new knowledge, although the subject may benefit incidentally.

Utilitarianism, utilitarian reasoning

The theory that what is right depends on the consequences; the end justifies the means; the right decision is determined by balancing risks and benefits.

Virtue

A character trait or disposition to be a good person.

Index